Feel Better
Naturally

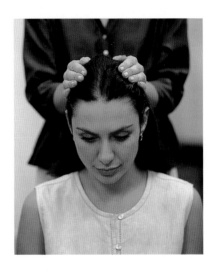

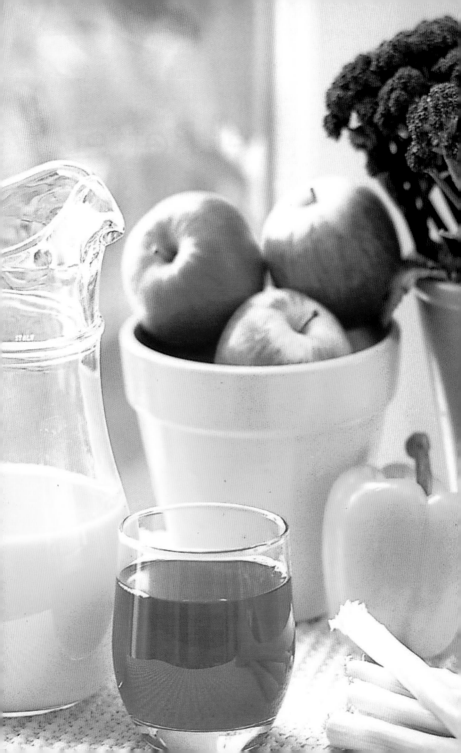

Feel Better
Naturally

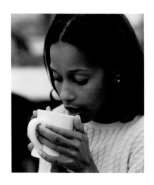

250 tips for feeling great
and performing better:
the complete guide to
health, harmony and simple
ways to stay on top of life

detox, tonics, soothers, rubs,
gargles, foot baths, massage,
comfort food, yoga, relaxers,
compresses, infusions,
reflexology, and more

Raje Airey and Tracey Kelly

southwater

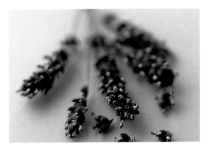

This edition is published by Southwater

Southwater is an imprint of
Anness Publishing Ltd
Hermes House, 88–89 Blackfriars Road
London SE1 8HA
tel. 020 7401 2077; fax 020 7633 9499
www.southwaterbooks.com; info@anness.com

© Anness Publishing Ltd 2005

UK agent: The Manning Partnership Ltd
6 The Old Dairy, Melcombe Road
Bath BA2 3LR
tel. 01225 478444; fax 01225 478440
sales@manning-partnership.co.uk

UK distributor: Grantham Book Services Ltd
Isaac Newton Way, Alma Park Industrial Estate
Grantham, Lincs NG31 9SD
tel. 01476 541080; fax 01476 541061
orders@gbs.tbs-ltd.co.uk

North American agent/distributor:
National Book Network
4501 Forbes Boulevard, Suite 200,
Lanham, MD 20706
tel. 301 459 3366; fax 301 429 5746
www.nbnbooks.com

Australian agent/distributor:
Pan Macmillan Australia
Level 18, St Martins Tower, 31 Market St,
Sydney, NSW 2000
tel. 1300 135 113; fax 1300 135 103
customer.service@macmillan.com.au

New Zealand agent/distributor:
David Bateman Ltd, 30 Tarndale Grove
Off Bush Road, Albany, Auckland
tel. (09) 415 7664; fax (09) 415 8892

A CIP catalogue record for this book is
available from the British Library.

Publisher: Joanna Lorenz
Editorial Director: Helen Sudell
Executive Editor: Joanne Rippin
Project Editors: Sue Barraclough, Caroline
Davison, Melanie Halton, Simona Hill, Ann
Kay & Catherine Stuart
Designers: Jester Designs, Lilian Lindblom,
Adelle Morris, Ian Sandhom & Lisa Tai
Photographers: Sue Atkinson, Martin Brigdale,
Sarah Cuttle, John Freeman, Michelle Garrett,
Christine Hanscomb, John Heseltine, Amanda
Heywood, Janine Hosegood, Alistair Hughes,
Andrea Jones, Don Last, William Lingwood, Liz
McAuley, Lucy Mason, Steve Moss, Thomas
Odulate, Debbie Patterson, Fiona Pragoff,
Craig Robertson, Simon Smith, Sam Stowell,
Stephen Swain & Steve Wooster
Text Editor: Jackie Matthews
Production Controller: Claire Rae

Previously published in five separate volumes,
*50 Natural Ways to Cure a Headache, 50 Natural
Ways to Relieve a Cold, 50 Natural Ways to
Relieve a Hangover, 50 Natural Ways
to Better Breathing* by Raje Airey &
50 Natural Ways to Relieve PMS by Tracey Kelly

10 9 8 7 6 5 4 3 2 1

Publisher's note:
The treatments in this book are safe to use in
the manner in which they are described.
They are not intended as a substitute for any
medicines prescribed by your doctor. If you
are taking prescribed medication, you should
always check with your doctor first before
trying other treatments.

contents

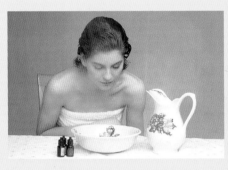

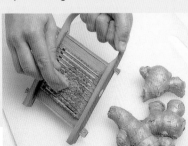

contents

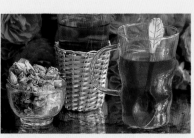

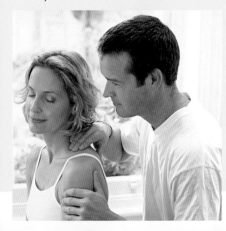

contents

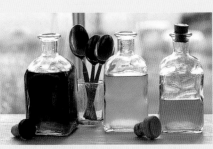

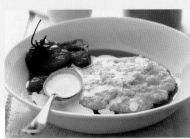

contents

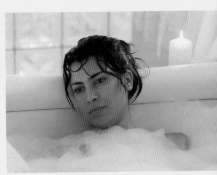

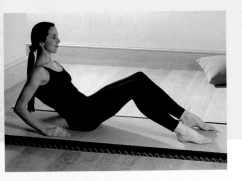

contents

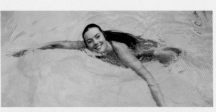

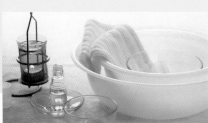

introduction

From time to time even the fittest of us are knocked back by an ailment that makes us feel wretched. It can be something as common as a cold or a headache, or a chest complaint that impairs our breathing. Women affected by premenstrual problems suffer an extra burden. And most of us, at least on occasion, experience the negative after-effects of drinking more alcohol than is good for us.

When thus afflicted, it's more than likely that we will reach for a bottle of painkillers or proprietary treatments to numb the pain. Yet what we could be doing is using safe, natural and effective methods to manage the problem and reduce its side effects. You can even use diet and exercise to avoid getting ill in the first place, building up your body's defences so that poor health is less likely to occur.

In this book you will find a truly holistic approach to overcoming common ailments and generating better health. It is packed with hundreds of simple and accessible treatments, including healing herbs, body-balancing foods, pain-easing exercises and gentle, mind-soothing therapies, as well as general dietary advice and excellent tips on how to curb our "fight or flight" response to stress and discomfort.

Headaches and migraines are caused by a number of factors, some of which – like tension, dehydration, illness, poor posture and diet – can be avoided. *Ease A Headache* suggests many different ways to overcome a headache quickly, or, better still, to avoid one altogether if you are prone to them. You'll find dozens of gentle, relaxing treatments designed to tackle pain quickly and effectively.

A cold can attack at any time, especially if your immune system is at a low ebb, and can be surprisingly debilitating in its effect, leaving body and spirit feeling battered. If you know how to deal with a cold as soon as it appears, you'll be better

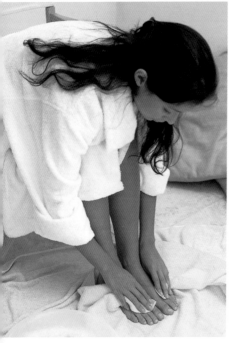

▲ *Taking care of every part of your body will help to boost all-round health.*

equipped to resist infection. What's more, if you know how to build up your immune system, you'll find that you are less vulnerable even when everyone else around you is falling like the proverbial fly. In *Beat a Cold* there are lots of comforting remedies and sound advice to make you feel better and stay that way.

Sometimes we seem to go out of our way to make ourselves ill. Not intentionally, of course, but as a by-product of having a really good time. Fortunately, *Lift a Hangover* is devoted to ways of getting over that horrible "morning after" feeling and quickly moving on from it. From detoxing juices and restorative, vitamin-rich foods to soothing and sensual touch-based therapies, you'll discover scores of terrific pick-me-ups.

Premenstrual syndrome (PMS) affects most women at some time. For some it is an occasional problem, for others it is a serious encumbrance. Whenever it strikes, things will improve immediately if you begin to understand the hormonal changes taking place in your body and work with them to take control, allowing you to get on with your life. *Relieve PMS* contains an astonishing array of symptom-easers, including exercise, supplements, diet and massage.

Breathing difficulties may result from a chronic respiratory condition such as asthma, or they may be a temporary imposition due to a cold

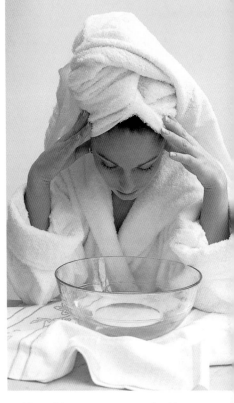

▲ *Many of the treatments prescribed here require very little effort to put into practice.*

or flu. In addition to respiratory remedies for clearing the airways, *Breathe Easier* includes treatments and routines for improving lung capacity as well as ways to avoid situations likely to aggravate breathing.

With this book as a handy guide, you'll be well on your way to feeling a whole lot better in both the short and the long term. It is simply a matter of identifying those treatments that will suit you best, and incorporating these measures into your lifestyle.

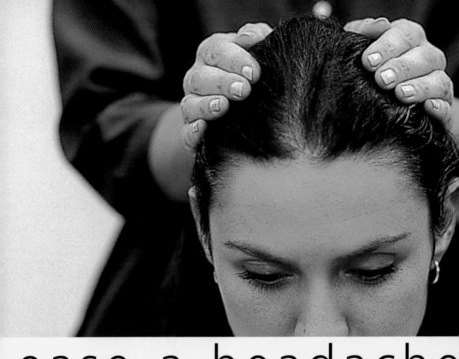

ease a headache

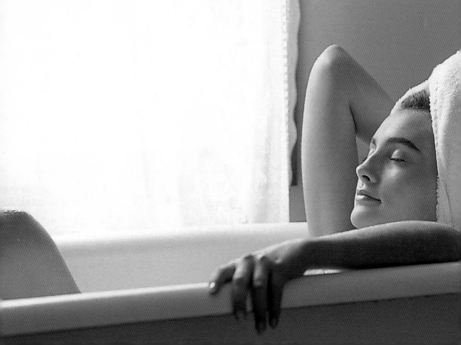

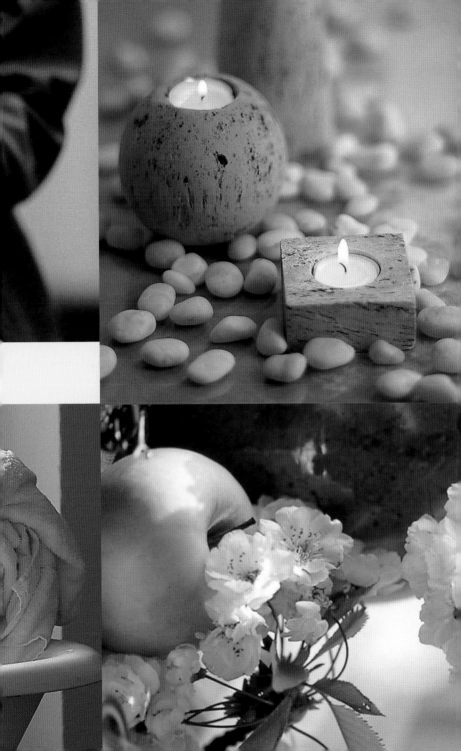

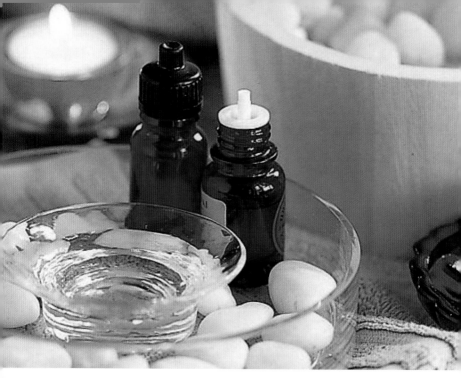

how to cure a headache

Almost everyone knows what it is like to have a headache. It is thought that more than 90 per cent of the population will have experienced a headache at one time or another, and unfortunately for many people they are almost a routine part of life.

There are hundreds of different causes of headaches, both psychological and physiological, and many different types of headache, ranging in severity from a crippling migraine which may last several days to a hangover headache which can clear up in a few hours. In some cases, headaches may indicate a major disorder such as a brain tumour or a life-threatening illness such as meningitis, but this is extremely rare.

Most headaches seen by the family doctor are known as "benign recurring headaches"; the vast majority of these are described as "tension headaches".

muscle restriction
Tension headaches are so-called because they are usually caused by some type of physical tension in the muscles of the shoulders, neck and head, and by constriction or congestion of the blood vessels in the head. The pain typically arises from the base of the skull (occiput) and extends up over the back of the head to the forehead and temples. The pain results from the continuous, partial contraction of muscles attached to the scalp and can affect the whole head.

Some people wake up with a headache, which then lasts all day with varying degrees of severity, ranging from a general dull ache to sudden jabbing pains in a particular spot. Other people experience this type of headache as a feeling of pressure, like a tight band around the head, or as a persistent throbbing. Although tension headaches are not associated with visual disturbance, many sufferers dislike bright light and find it hard to concentrate.

migraines

Many regular headache sufferers describe their condition as "having a migraine". However, a migraine is a specific medical condition and is not the same as an everyday tension headache. Migraines are a fairly common neurological disorder, with three times as many women as men suffering. Many women's migraines occur premenstrually and are linked to hormonal imbalances.

The severe pain of a migraine headache is thought to be caused by the dilation (swelling up) of the blood vessels in the head, causing a disturbance in the flow of blood to the brain. This follows a brief period of constriction of the vessels which partly

accounts for the visual disturbances (known as "aura") that many people experience prior to the headache. Migraines cause chemical changes in the body and typical symptoms include aversion to light (photophobia), nausea, vomiting and diarrhoea. The headache itself is often one-sided and is marked by severe pain in the forehead or temples, or rising up from the back of the neck. A migraine attack can last up to 72 hours and becomes extremely debilitating. It can take a day or two after an attack to get back to normal.

bouts of pain

Cluster headaches are often confused with migraine as the severe pain tends to be centred around the eye area and is typically one-sided. These headaches occur in bouts during a 1–2 month period. In an attack, the headache will come on suddenly and

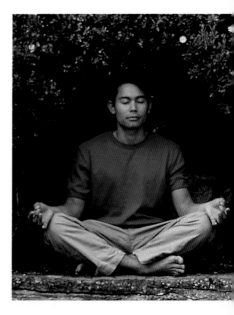

how to cure a headache / **15**

last up to an hour. Several attacks may be experienced in a day, often waking the sufferer from sleep, or causing them to pace about as the pain is so intense. Cluster headaches are less common than migraines; they rarely occur in anyone under 30 and most sufferers are men. Drinking alcohol during a bout can bring on an attack.

a symptom of another illness

Other types of headache arise as secondary symptoms of problems elsewhere in the body. This may include mechanical injuries, such as whiplash or head injuries, or general wear and tear on the body, caused by failing eyesight, poor posture, or arthritis in the neck, for instance. Similarly, headaches associated with premenstrual syndrome (PMS), high blood pressure, blocked sinuses, inflammation of the middle ear and viral infections are also fairly common.

headache triggers

Most headaches do not come out of the blue, but are triggered by certain factors. Migraines, cluster and tension headaches are typically linked to stress, overwork and negative emotional states such as worry, anxiety, depression and held-in anger and resentment. After stress, food allergies and/or intolerances are one of the most common causes of migraine and tension headaches. Certain foods, such as red wine, cheese and chocolate, are well-known triggers. Others include low blood sugar, caffeine withdrawal, lack of sleep and toxicity in the body, caused by poor digestion or over-indulgence in sugar and alcohol, for instance. Long-distance driving, too much sun, changes in the weather and sensitivities to environmental triggers, such as perfume, car exhaust fumes, cigarette smoke and paint fumes, can also play a part.

nature's remedies

Conventional treatment for a headache is standard painkillers, either available on prescription for migraine and severe headaches, or over-the-counter for everyday tension headaches. The drugs often combine painkillers, such as aspirin or paracetamol, with other drugs which have a sedative, antispasmodic action. Because these drugs are so common and easily available, we tend to think they are harmless and that we can take them every day. While these drugs have their place, they also have many potentially harmful side effects, particularly if taken on a regular basis. It is believed that many people are addicted to painkillers, and that many headaches are caused as the result of taking too many pills. For this reason, increasing numbers of people are turning to natural medicine as they look for effective treatments which are non-habit forming and non-toxic.

This section contains information and ideas for how to treat headaches without using drugs. In natural medicine, pain is seen as the body's way of telling you that something is

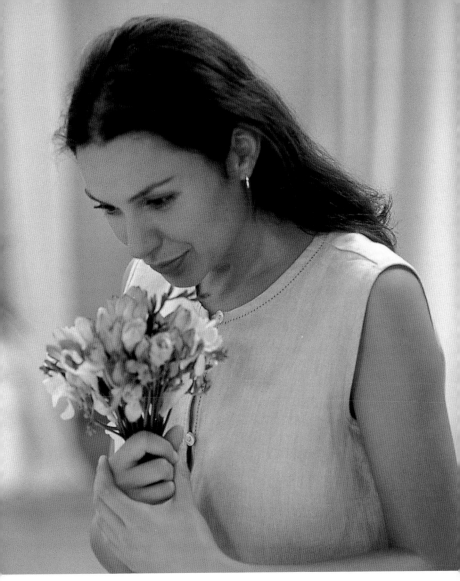

wrong; it has a protective function, acting as an "early warning system". Consequently, many of the treatments are based on dealing with the underlying cause of the pain and recognizing the importance of diet, lifestyle and psychological factors. Natural remedies can be used to help

▲ *Most people appreciate the soft and subtle scent of flowers. Their gentle perfume can help relieve a headache.*

the body work through its own healing process with minimum discomfort. Use it as a guide to find a treatment that is just right for you.

headache treatments

The headache treatments featured in this section are based on holistic principles. This means they have an underlying assumption that an individual's good health depends on a balance between physical, mental, emotional and spiritual well-being.The treatments are drawn from a wide variety of natural-healing traditions; some of these practices have been used around the world for centuries as aids for relieving headaches as well as avoiding them by generally promoting health and well-being. They are all based on therapeutic techniques which help to stimulate the body's own natural healing ability, and include hands-on therapies such as massage, shiatsu and reflexology as well as treatments based on herbal remedies, aromatherapy and nutrition. There are also treatments to relieve headache-inducing stress and tension, such as meditation and yoga, and subtle energy healing methods using reiki, crystals and colour. Every headache sufferer is sure to find here a remedy that is suited to their personal makeup.

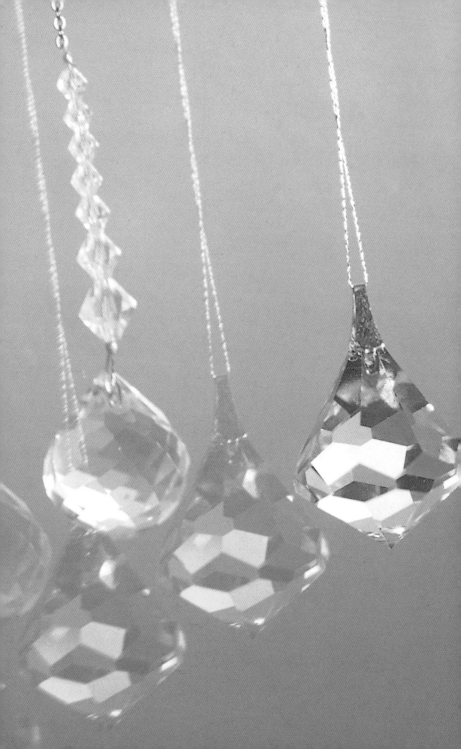

1 refreshing water

The body of a healthy adult is made up of about 75 per cent water. Water is vital for life, yet many common health problems, such as headaches, are linked with dehydration.

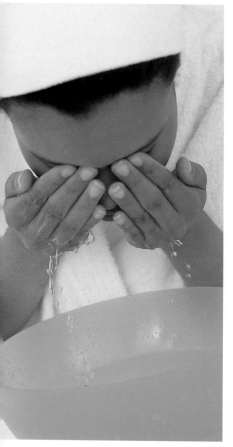

▲ Water is revitalizing and refreshing and an excellent panacea for a headache.

Start the day with a glass of water. This flushes out your kidneys and detoxifies your system. Water is best drunk half an hour before eating and between meals, to allow for the flushing action and to avoid interfering with the body's digestive processes.

At the first sign of a headache, drink a couple of glasses of water. Often this is enough for it to lift without the need for further treatment. Add a slice of lemon for a refreshing tang and a burst of vitamin C to kick-start the liver. Drinking water when stressed or anxious also helps to keep your body fluids flowing smoothly and can help to calm you down.

To dispel headaches brought on by eyestrain, try splashing the eyes and forehead with warm and then cold water. This stimulates the circulation and refreshes tired eyes.

KEEP HYDRATED
Alcohol, tea, coffee and fizzy drinks are diuretics; for every drink it is recommended to drink at least one glass of water to counter its effect.

2

walking & posture

If you suffer from tension headaches, make walking an everyday part of life. Walking is an excellent stress-busting form of exercise, but to get the best benefit you need good posture.

When we are stressed, the body responds by producing extra adrenaline as its "fight or flight" mechanism comes into force. If this adrenaline is not used, it overloads the system and gets stored in the body, creating tense, tight muscles, which leads to headaches. No matter what your age, weight or physical build, regular walking will help to improve your general health.

Regular activity

You can build walking into your normal routine so that it becomes an everyday activity. Find opportunities for walking in regular activities: take the stairs instead of the elevator; walk to work or the shops rather than use the car; or use a manual lawnmower to mow the grass.

When you have more time, your daily routine will have prepared you for more strenuous activity. A day's hike over spectacular hills or perhaps a more gentle afternoon stroll in the countryside will disperse stresses built up over a long working week.

Good posture

As you walk, lead with your head and allow the whole of your body to lengthen, so that your arms are free to move and your legs can follow.

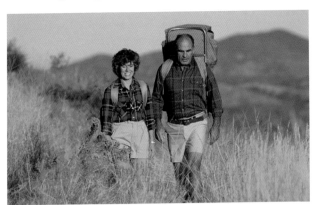

◄ Make walking a sociable and enjoyable part of your regular exercise routine. Hiking enables you to experience beautiful locations that are otherwise inaccessible.

3 easy neck stretches

Many tension headaches begin with a feeling of pressure in the head or at the base of the neck. A few simple stretches can help to relieve this muscular tension before the headache kicks in.

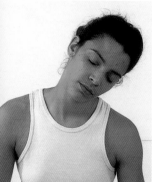

head and neck stretch

1 Turn the head to one side, then slowly rotate it in a semicircular movement, letting the chin drop down across the chest. Repeat in the opposite direction.

2 For an extra stretch, slowly stretch your head down to one side, feeling the pull in the neck muscles. Use your hands as a lever to make this side stretch more effective. Place one hand under your chin and the other on top of your head; as you stretch sideways, exert a steady pressure with both hands, but be careful not to pull or tug your head. Change hands and repeat on the other side.

face work-out

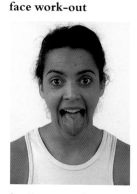

Another area where you hold a lot of tension is the face. This simple exercise is excellent for stretching the delicate facial muscles to release tension. To do it, find a quiet spot where you are unobserved. Open your mouth as wide as possible and push out your tongue. At the same time, open your eyes into as wide a stare as you can manage. Hold for a moment or two then relax. Repeat a couple of times.

4 relaxing yoga positions

Yoga relaxes the muscles, slows the breath and brings stillness to the mind, making it a useful therapy for treating stress-related disorders. These two poses can be undertaken by anyone.

standing bend ›
Place a headrest on a stool. Stand with your feet parallel and hip width apart. Breathe out and bend forwards from the hips slowly. Rest your arms over your head on the stool and relax for 1–2 minutes.

lying flat ▾
Lie on a flat surface, with your legs and arms releasing out to the sides. Use a cushion if you feel more comfortable. Close your eyes and relax for 10–15 minutes.

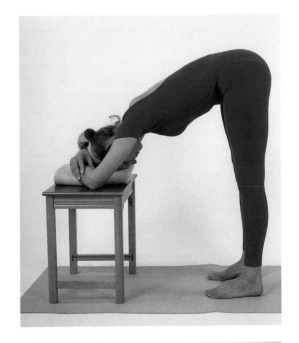

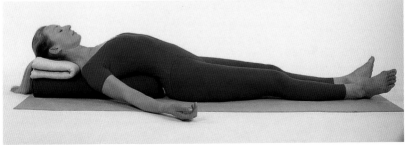

5 healthy eating

Food fuels the body. Frequent headaches may be linked to a poor diet, so it is worth spending time preparing meals from good quality, fresh ingredients rather than using convenience foods.

A well-balanced diet is rich in fibre, vitamins and minerals; this means eating plenty of fresh fruit and vegetables, wholegrains such as rice, millet and barley, and wholegrain bread and cereals. For protein, eat a little lean meat, poultry, fish, cheese, nuts and soya products.

B-complex vitamins
Having enough of the B-complex vitamins is necessary for the healthy functioning of the nervous system. They get used up more rapidly when we are under stress. Studies have shown that niacin (B_3) can help prevent and ease the severity of migraines. The best natural sources are in liver, kidney, lean meat, wholegrains, brewer's yeast, wheat germ, fish, eggs, roasted peanuts, the white meat of poultry, avocados, dates, figs and prunes.

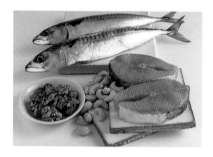

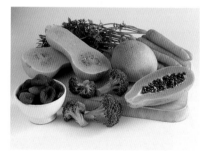

▲ *Choose organic products as these are free from potentially harmful toxic residues.*

HEALTHY CHOICES
If you are prone to headaches, cut down on your intake of processed foods, sugar, salt, refined carbohydrates, tea, coffee, fizzy drinks and alcohol.

Many common foods contain chemicals that can trigger neural and blood vessel changes in the brain, causing migraines or severe headaches in susceptible people. Common migraine triggers are chocolate, citrus fruits, cheese, coffee, bacon and alcohol, particularly red wine.

6 quick-fix snacks

Many headaches are caused by a low blood-sugar level. As your energy level drops, don't be tempted to go for an instant fix with caffeine or sugar; instead choose healthy snacks.

There are many steps you can take to help break an unhealthy cycle. Avoid the temptation to snack unhealthily or to miss meals and "eat on the run". A few nuts or seeds or a piece of fresh fruit is a good substitute for a chocolate bar or bag of crisps (potato chips).

healthy food rules

Eating little and often is a good habit to cultivate. Eat regular light meals, based on fresh, whole ingredients, every 3–4 hours. This will help to stabilize your blood sugar level and prevent excessive energy swings. You should feel better and notice an improvement in your headaches.

Monitor your intake of caffeinated drinks and limit yourself to no more than one or two cups of tea or coffee a day. There are many replacements, such as herbal teas and cereal coffees made from barley, rye, chicory or acorns for instance, which are available in good health stores. Replace sugar with a little fructose (fruit sugar) or honey, either of which is preferable to an artificial sweetener or refined sugar.

▼ *Complex carbohydrates are the best source of energy. Nuts are filling and release energy slowly.*

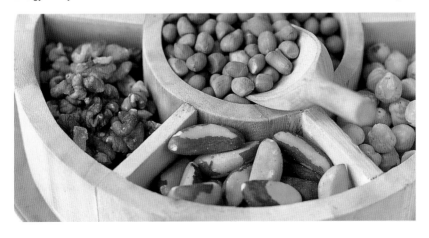

7 food intolerance

Most migraine sufferers are aware that certain foods and drinks can trigger an attack. Frequent headaches may also be a symptom of widespread and recognized food allergies or intolerances.

Food intolerance is when the body becomes hypersensitive to certain foods; the immune system perceives the substance as harmful, and sets off a chain reaction in the body which produces various symptoms, including sneezing, itchy rashes, sinus problems, lethargy, an uncomfortable bloated feeling and headaches. The onset of food intolerance can occur at any age and to a substance that was previously tolerated. The only way of finding out if you have a food intolerance is to eliminate the suspect food(s) from your diet, one at a time, and see whether your symptoms disappear.

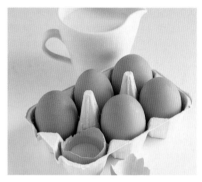

▲ Try cutting out cow's milk or eggs to help your headache symptoms.

Common offenders include products made from cow's milk, wheat, corn, yeast, eggs, nuts and shellfish.

plan ahead
If you think you may have a food intolerance and want to try an elimination diet, make sure you plan ahead so that you don't run out of suitable foods. Base your diet on fresh foods and do not skip meals. Avoid eating out, or if you do, choose plainly cooked dishes. Always check the labels on any manufactured foods, in case they contain the foods that you want to eliminate.

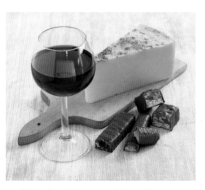

▲ Red wine, cheese and chocolate can bring on migraines for some people.

8 fresh fruit fusion

Toxicity in the body is one of the principal causes of headaches. Often this is the result of digestive problems such as constipation and/or the absorption of incompletely digested foods.

A sedentary lifestyle combined with a diet low in fibre and water and high in processed foods and caffeinated drinks makes constipation a common health problem. Additionally, regular use of antibiotics and other drugs, alcohol and/or a high intake of sugar can lead to inflammation of the walls of the small intestine, causing intestinal permeability or a 'leaky gut'. This means that toxic waste is reabsorbed through the intestinal wall back into the bloodstream, causing headaches, fatigue, skin problems and bad breath.

To improve digestion, increase your daily intake of fibre–rich foods, such as raw fruit and vegetables, brown rice and wholegrains. You should also increase your fluid intake. Filtered water is a must, but for a detox include fresh fruit and vegetable juices.

apple, red cabbage and fennel fusion
All fresh juices have a cleansing effect on the digestive system and are gently laxative. This is a surprisingly delicious combination – fennel has a distinctive aniseed flavour that blends well with both fruit and vegetables. To prepare this recipe, you will need half a small red cabbage, half a fennel bulb, two apples, plus 15ml/1 tbsp freshly squeezed lemon juice. Roughly slice the cabbage and fennel and quarter the apples. Using a juice extractor, juice the vegetables and fruit. Add the lemon juice to the mixture and stir to combine. Serve immediately in a glass.

▾ *Always buy firm, fresh-looking fennel and use within a couple of days. If left too long, it will discolour and turn fibrous.*

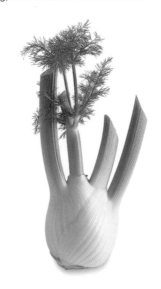

9

During sex, the body relaxes, easing muscular tension and dissolving energy blocks, which are often the source of headaches. It is one of the best natural therapies there is.

10 get a good night's rest

Sleep is one of nature's great healers. During sleep the cells of the body renew and repair themselves. Sleep deprivation can lead to all kinds of physical and emotional problems including headaches.

Sleeplessness is a common response to stress as your mind and body cannot let go enough to give you the rest you need. If you have headaches caused by stress, learning to switch off and relax is essential for promoting restful sleep. Make sure you have a healthy diet, take regular exercise and have a calming routine to wind down before bedtime.

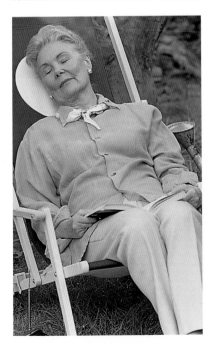

SLEEP DO'S AND DON'TS
• Get plenty of fresh air and exercise on a regular basis.
• Don't sleep in late, but get up early and get yourself moving.
• Avoid drinking caffeinated drinks such as cola, tea and coffee at bedtime. A herbal tea or a warm, milky drink is a better alternative.
• Sleep in a well-ventilated room, preferably with the window open.
• Avoid heavy meals late at night.
• Essential oils such as lavender, chamomile and marjoram all have sedative properties. Add a couple of drops of one of them to a warm bath before bedtime, or else put a couple of drops on to a paper tissue and place under the pillow.
• Hops can be dried and used to fill a "sleep cushion" for the bed. Alternatively, they can be brewed and made into a tea, to be drunk before you go to bed.

◀ If you can't sleep at night but find yourself falling asleep in the middle of the day, it's time to rethink your daily routine.

For animal lovers, keeping a pet can be **therapeutic**. If you feel a headache coming on, take the **dog** for a walk or sit and stroke your **cat** – you may find that the headache disappears.

12 laughter as medicine

Laughter is nature's tonic. It eases muscle tension, deepens breathing, improves circulation and releases headache-relieving endorphins to the brain to give you a natural "high".

If you feel you spend too much time working and not enough time having fun, or too much time on your own and not enough time with friends or family, try to redress the balance. Research shows there is a strong link between happiness and good health, so balance the stress of daily life by spending time regularly with friends and family.

▾ *Laughter makes the world look brighter.*

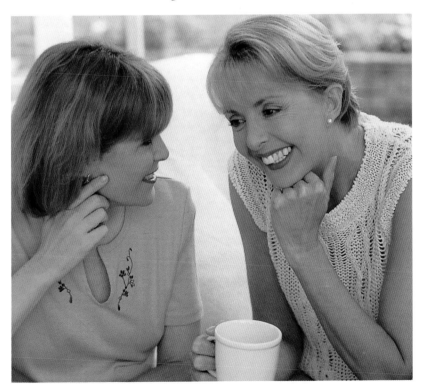

13

rose quartz stress buster

Crystal healing is one of the most effective ways of allowing trapped energy to release safely. Rose quartz is particularly useful for removing blocked emotional stress which often leads to a headache.

emotional release

Unresolved emotional stress can become locked in any part of the body, but often accumulates around the neck and shoulders, where the restricted flow of energy results in a headache. To release such stress rapidly and safely, lie down on your back, face upwards, and place small rose quartz stones on the slightly raised bumps to the sides of the forehead. You may need to tape the stones in place. To begin the release, recall the stressful event. The process will be complete when you feel a change of emotion or a return of equilibrium. Placing a grounding stone by the feet and a balancing stone at the heart or solar plexus chakra may also help.

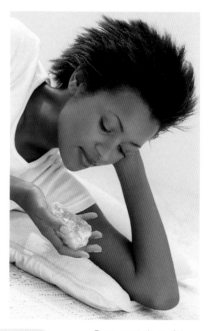

▲ Rose quartz is useful for reducing any build-up of emotional stress and tension which can trigger a headache. Keeping some rose quartz at your bedside can also be effective as an aid to restful sleep.

CRYSTAL CLEANSING
Because crystals act as energy transmitters, it is important to keep them clean. Before using them for healing they should always be washed in salt water. Ideally they should be left overnight, covered in salted water; the salt has a purifying action, helping to draw out any negativity which is being "held" in the stones. Always pour the water away.

14 headache healing spell

Try this ancient incantation to cure all types of
headache. Before you make the spell, find a
suitable tree to bury it under – ash, birch, juniper,
orange and cedar trees all have healing powers.

you will need
gold candle and match
gold pen
15cm (6in) square of natural paper
knife
lime
gold cord
15cm (6in) square of orange cloth
spade

1 Light the candle and invite your
guardian angel or spirit helper to
support the healing. Make up your
own words, or say the following:

*I light this flame to honour
your presence and ask you to
hear this prayer.*

2 Write your name clearly with the
pen on the paper, at the same time
visualizing a protective bubble of
health and well-being surrounding
you. Keep yourself focused.

3 Cut the lime lengthways into two.
Fold the paper three times and place
it between the two lime halves. Bind
the lime halves together with gold
cord, while saying the following
invocation (prayer):

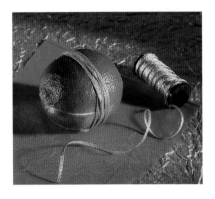

*Powers of lime,
Health is mine,
Cleanse the body,
Cleanse the mind,
Spirit pure,
Fill my being with health,
With health,
With health.*

4 Place the bound lime in the orange
cloth and bind the cloth with gold
cord. Blow out the candle and say
farewell to your higher self, guardian
angel or spirit helper.

5 Bury the parcel in the earth under
your chosen tree. Ask the tree to help
you return to good health and thank
the tree.

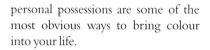

15 blue colour therapy

Colours can affect our mood and we can tap into this power to use colour for healing purposes. Blue is one of the best colours for calming and soothing frayed nerves.

To ease a tension headache, look for colours which have a calming and cooling effect on the mind and emotions. When you need rest and healing, blue is a good colour to choose. Blue is the colour of the seas and skies and is associated with peace and tranquillity. Soft and soothing blue is a perfect antidote to the stresses, strains and tensions of modern living.

You can work with colour in a variety of ways. The clothes you wear, the decor of your room and your personal possessions are some of the most obvious ways to bring colour into your life.

changing the environment
Bathe yourself in coloured light using coloured films in combination with a free-standing spotlight. To do this, place a sheet of coloured film over the light, making sure that it is not touching the hot bulb. Turn off all the other lights and turn on the spotlight. If it is daytime, draw the curtains or blinds. Sit in the path of the spotlight's ray and bathe in the coloured light for an instant, on-the-spot therapy.

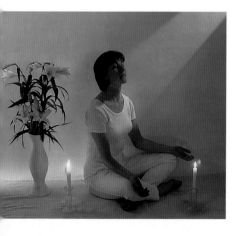

COLOUR CHOICES
You may have noticed that your preference for particular colours varies over time. Start paying attention to which colours attract and which ones repel you. It may mean that you need more of the ones you are attracted to, and a bit less of the others.

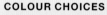

◀ Blue is restful on the eye and is excellent for slowing things down.

16 green colour therapy

In the spectrum of colours, green lies centrally between red and blue. Green can have a balancing, harmonizing effect. The green of the natural world is nourishing to the spirits.

Take a walk in a leafy green forest and feel the colour green refresh and revitalize you. A walk in the country, taking in fresh air, has the same effect. For headaches arising from nervous exhaustion and debility, green is a good colour to work with. Green is the colour of harmony; it is an excellent tonic for the nerves and helps to restore stability when you are out of balance. Green is all around us in so many tonal values. Light, vibrant green in particular has an uplifting effect on the spirit and is useful when you are feeling depressed.

colour vibration

One way of treating yourself is to have a selection of coloured silks which you can use to wrap yourself in. By wrapping coloured silk around your body, you envelop yourself in pure colour vibration. Choose the colour to which you feel most attracted for your treatment. Turquoise has a soothing and calming effect on the central nervous system.

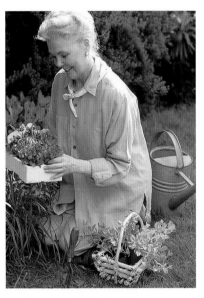

▲ When you are feeling drained, spend some time in a quiet park, garden or green fields and notice the effect on your energy levels.

STRESS BUSTER
If you don't have a large piece of cloth, a small, green silk square placed behind your head in a chair can relieve tension and pressure.

17 relax your body

Relaxation is as important for your health and well-being as exercise and a nutritious diet. If you do not switch off from the tensions of everyday life, you are more likely to suffer frequent headaches.

Breathing is something you do unconsciously, but when you are relaxed and calm your breathing pattern is different from when you are tense, anxious or negative. At times of great tension and stress, breathing is usually irregular and shallow, and does not completely fulfil your need for oxygen. If you learn to control your breathing it will help you to stay relaxed even in the most tense or stressful situations.

breathe deeply
Working with the breath is one of the best ways to relax both mind and body. This technique is often used at the end of yoga or exercise sessions. Here is a simple breath control strategy that you can practise at any time. Learning to focus your attention on just your breathing and nothing else will enhance your body awareness and control and help to make you feel calm and centred.

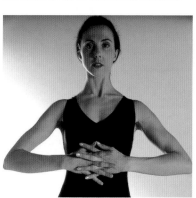

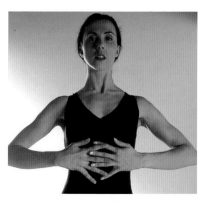

1 Place your hands with your palms under your chest, on your ribs, and your fingers loosely interlocked. Inhale slowly and continuously through your nose, to a count of four. Do not strain, keep yourself relaxed.

2 As you inhale, concentrate on allowing your ribs to expand laterally: your fingers should gently part. Don't let your ribs jut forward. Exhale slowly, expelling all the breath from the lungs, then repeat.

18 relax your mind

A short meditation break in the day will help your mind to unwind and help you return to your activities with a clear head. Meditating at night will help you to relax and prepare for sleep.

visualization exercise

Sit down in a comfortable spot where you won't be disturbed. Close your eyes and allow your mind to drift to a pleasant, peaceful place. A special place where you can relax … completely. A safe … secure … place … where nothing can ever bother you. It may be a place that you know … or one that you imagine. Perhaps a garden … or a place in the countryside … or maybe a room. But it is a place where you feel safe and able to let go … completely … a place that is unique and special to you.

When you are in your place… notice the light: is it bright, natural or dim? Notice also the temperature level … hot, warm or cool? Be aware of the colours that surround you … the shapes … and textures … the familiar objects that make that place special.

Continue to relax in your special place … enjoying the sounds … the smells … the atmosphere … with nobody wanting anything from you … just you in your special place where you can truly relax.

To end the meditation, slowly

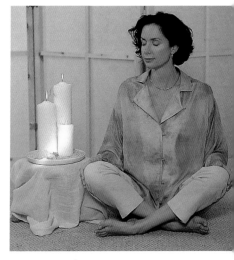

▲ *Candlelit rooms help create the right mood for meditation.*

bring your attention back to the room. When you are ready, open your eyes.

CHANGE YOUR BRAINWAVES
Meditation is one of the best forms of relaxation there is; in meditation, the brain-wave pattern changes to relaxed alpha waves, similar to the pattern shown in sleep.

19 protective visualization

Tap into the creative power of your imagination to increase your health and well-being and help remove the stress that causes headaches. Creative visualization is simple to learn and effective.

A lot of the stress of daily living comes from trying to satisfy the needs, demands and expectations of others. When the pressure becomes too much, it is easy to react by snapping angrily or by swallowing feelings of resentment and hostility. This is a classic scenario for a thumping headache. To protect yourself from outside pressure, try this visualization which involves creating a protective bubble or shield around yourself.

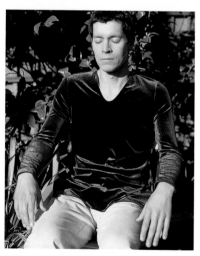

▲ "Thinking yourself well" has many beneficial effects.

calm and clarity

Sit comfortably, close your eyes and imagine yourself in the kind of stressful situation that typically leads to a headache. Picture yourself and any other people who may be involved. Now notice a slight shimmer of light between yourself and the other people … a protective bubble around you. Learn to believe that this bubble only allows positive and helpful energies to reach you and reflects any negativity back to its source … leaving you free to get on with your life feeling calm and inwardly strong.

While you are in your bubble of light, imagine talking to someone who has been causing pressure to build. See yourself communicating with that person in a calm and clear way until they understand the position. Next, find unhelpful emotions such as past resentments and hurts and imagine pushing them out through the bubble where they can no longer limit or harm you. As you finish the visualization, remind yourself that the bubble stays with you, protecting you. Use this technique next time you feel a headache coming on.

20 gentle candlelight

Practically all headaches feel worse if you are surrounded by harsh bright light. The warm soft glow of candlelight creates a comforting and soothing ambience. Use it to help you unwind.

choosing candles

To help a headache, combine some aroma and colour therapy and choose candles with healing scents and hues. Simple white candles are effective, or look for pale, soft colours, such as pinks and mauves which have a healing effect on the emotions. Avoid large candles in shades of vibrant red and orange, acid green and yellow or dark purple and black.

soothing aromas

Scent is largely a matter of personal preference, but when you have a headache sickly sweet smells such as vanilla or heavy scents such as musk are probably best avoided. Some people like light floral scents, while others may prefer hints of fresh citrus. Sandalwood is also a good choice; this fragrance is traditionally used as a therapeutic aid to meditation, as it helps the mind to relax. Frankincense is another scent which is used in meditation; it has a calming effect on the nerves and slows down the breathing. If you don't like perfumed candles but would like to use scent, you could burn incense sticks or vaporize essential oils instead.

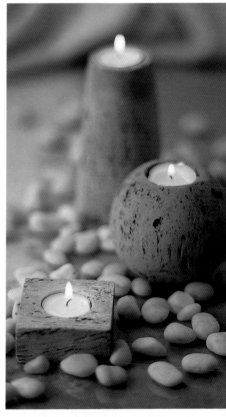

▲ *A warm and uncluttered room is a good place to relax by candlelight. Make sure that the candles are in a suitable container to protect your furniture from hot candle wax.*

21 clear the clutter

Too much paraphernalia in our lives makes us overburdened, depleting our energy and leaving us open to illness of all kinds. Keeping your space clutter-free keeps the energy pathways clear.

Books, papers and toys left lying around, untidy cupboards or work-spaces, anything that's kept "just in case", and any unfinished tasks or jobs which need to be done are all examples of clutter. When you start to accumulate junk, it's a fact that you will always add to it. Having piles of debris lying around, and items wrongly filed or waiting to be put away, will eventually wear you down and hinder your movement around a room. Once a whole house becomes cluttered, the effect is debilitating and depressing, leading to illness. Notice the effect on your energy levels after you have had a good clear-out.

TASK LIST

Make a list of all the jobs that need doing and put them in order of priority; make a point of tackling something on your list each day.

• Go through your cupboards and have a clear out at least twice a year. Throw out anything that you are not using and no longer need.
• Don't forget to clear places like the loft, garden shed and cellar. They are typical dumping grounds for clutter.
• Always keep your desk and work area clear.
• Deal with correspondence quickly and don't let things lie in your in-tray for too long.
• If you find it difficult to throw things away, then ask a friend to help you. They won't have an emotional attachment to your things, and will be able to offer you a more objective opinion.

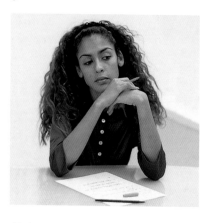

◄ *Make a list of any items you can sell, any jobs that need finishing or items that need mending, as you work through your space.*

healing homeopathy

Homeopathic remedies are prepared by diluting the original substance until what is left is a vibrational essence. These headache remedies stimulate the body to heal itself from within.

There are hundreds of remedies which are suitable for treating headaches, but below are some of the most widely available. Choose the remedy that most closely matches your symptoms. Take it three times a day in the 6C potency or once a day in the 30C potency until your symptoms have improved.

Belladonna for a throbbing, hammering headache that is worse at the temples, and the headache may be accompanied by fever.
Euphrasia for a headache accompanied by painful, watering eyes, where the sufferer is unable to bear bright light.

Hypericum for a pain that is lessened by bending the head backwards.
Nat. Mur for a migraine-type headache, which is preceded by misty vision or flickering lights in the eyes.
Nux Vomica to lessen the pain of a hangover headache.
Pulsatilla for a headache brought on by overwork, or associated with pre-menstrual tension or the menopause.
Silica for a headache that starts at the base of the neck and spreads up over the scalp, settling over the eyes.
Sulphur for a throbbing headache, which is improved when lying on the right and when gentle pressure is applied to the head.

▸ Homeopathic remedies are made from plant, mineral and animal substances, some of which are highly poisonous in their original form. Because the remedies are diluted many times they are safe to use and have no harmful side effects.

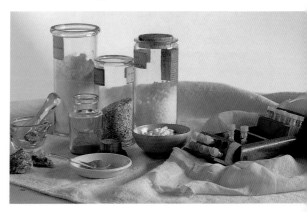

23 reiki headache treatment

Reiki is a form of Japanese spiritual healing whereby chi, or "life energy", is channelled, in the case of a headache treatment, through the practitioner's hands on to the head of the sufferer.

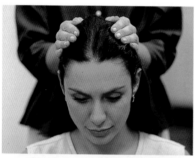

1 Stand behind your partner and place both (warm) hands firmly on the sides of the head at the back, with your fingers coming up on to the top of the head. This cradling action feels very supportive and helps to dispel tension rising from the neck, balancing energy in the brain. Hold the position for a few minutes.

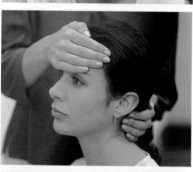

2 Move to the side, and place one hand firmly on the forehead and the other at the base of the skull. Reiki works by putting the hands in certain positions on the body and then allowing the healing energy to flow through them. The aim of the treatment is to dissolve energy blocks and rebalance the body.

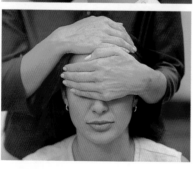

3 Finish by placing one hand lightly over the eyes and the other on top of the head. This is very relaxing. After giving healing, you should always wash your hands. The person receiving reiki should drink plenty of water after the treatment to help flush out toxins. A reiki treatment can bring rapid relief from a headache.

24 healing herb tub

Many of the remedies suggested in this book use plants. For quality and freshness, nothing beats growing your own. An attractive way of doing this is to plant up a container of healing herbs.

Use a large container to give the plants room to grow and site it in a sunny spot near the house for easy access.

you will need
Half-barrel
Bricks
Drainage material
Soilless compost (growing medium)
Sharp sand
Watering can

plants
Feverfew (*Tanacetum parthenium*)
Lavender (*Lavandula* 'Hidcote',
    L. stoechas)
Marjoram (*Origanum vulgare*
    'Variegatum')
Rosemary (*Rosmarinus officinalis*),
    prostrate and upright forms
Lemon balm (*Melissa officinalis*)

1 Rest the tub on a few bricks to raise it off the ground and promote better drainage. Cover the base with a layer of drainage material such as broken pots, broken polystyrene plant trays or horticultural grit. Almost fill the tub with a 50/50 mixture of compost and sharp sand.

2 Arrange the herbs, still in their pots, on the surface of the compost. When you are happy with the arrangement, make holes and plant them, firming the compost down and topping up if necessary. Leave a gap below the rim of the tub to allow for watering. Water the plants in well.

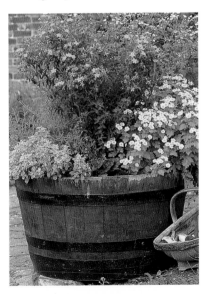

▼ *Keep the plants well trimmed and replace the top layer of compost annually. Feed regularly in the summer months.*

25

lavender &
rosemary oils

There are many essential oils which can help treat a headache, but two of the most popular and effective are lavender and rosemary, which are both from the same plant family.

Lavender is particularly good for headaches that are related to stress and tension, while rosemary is useful for ones brought on by mental fatigue and nervous exhaustion; either is useful for headaches associated with depression. A quick and convenient headache treatment is to mix a drop of either oil in a teaspoon of carrier oil, such as almond. Rub the mix into your temples. Or put a drop of neat oil on a handkerchief and inhale the aroma.

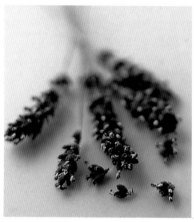

▲ Lavender has many healing properties. It is an excellent headache remedy as it is a natural analgesic.

▼ Rosemary helps to regulate blood pressure and can reduce pain.

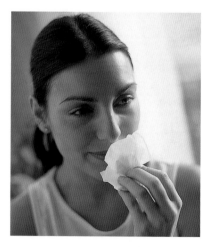

HOW OILS WORK
Inhalation is the fastest way of enjoying the benefits of aromatic oils, as nerve pathways lead directly from the lining of the nose to the brain, having an immediate effect on the central nervous system.

CAUTION: Do not use rosemary oil if you are pregnant or suffer from epilepsy.

26 soothing bath water

Make up this bubble bath mix and keep it on standby for when you need to relax at the end of a long, stressful day – it will ease a headache and promote restful sleep.

lavender bubble bath

The recipe uses dried lavender flowers as well as lavender oil for extra strength. The mixture will keep for several months in a cool, dark place.

you will need

medium-sized bottle of clear, mild,
   unscented shampoo
45ml/3 tbsp dried lavender flowers
5 drops lavender essential oil
wide-necked, screw-topped glass jar
fine sieve
glass or plastic jug (pitcher)
squeezable plastic bottle

1 Pour the shampoo, the lavender flowers and the lavender oil into the glass jar. Replace the lid and shake vigorously to mix all the ingredients thoroughly together.

2 Leave this mixture to stand in a warm place, such as a sunny windowsill, for up to two weeks, shaking and turning the jar occasionally. The lavender flowers will infuse the shampoo.

3 Strain off the lavender liquid into the jug and then pour it into the squeezable plastic bottle. Discard the dried lavender flowers.

▸ *Let the day's tensions melt away with the delicate fragrance of lavender. Lavender is a recognized cure-all for many common ailments, including tense, nervous headaches.*

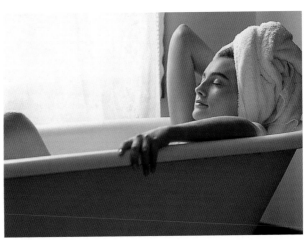

a relaxing atmosphere

Scenting the environment can soothe a headache and help you regain equilibrium quickly. Try using a vaporizer with a few drops of your favourite essential oil.

The bedroom and bathroom are both ideal places to relax, while the use of soft music, candles and essential oil burners is a popular way of creating a peaceful and soothing atmosphere. Essential oil burners have a small dish to hold water and a source of gentle heat underneath, often a night-light candle. The heat needs to be fairly low, but warm enough to heat up the water. A few drops of essential oil are added to the warm water, which then slowly evaporates, giving out its scent. Alternatively, oil drops can be added to a bowl of hot water if you do not have a burner.

Any of the following oils will help to create a relaxing atmosphere. Add two or three drops to a burner.

Clary Sage for stress and tension headaches.

Geranium for headaches caused by premenstrual syndrome.

Lavender for migraine and tension headaches.

Neroli for headaches caused by mental exertion.

Rose to soothe and calm the nerves.

Sweet Marjoram for headaches caused by anxiety and insomnia.

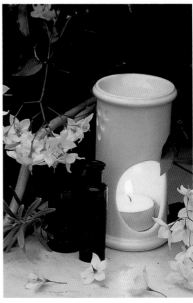

▲ *Essential oils help speed up the healing process. Use them as an aid to recovery, as well as to scent your room.*

BE PREPARED
Carry a small bottle of your favourite essential oil with you and try dabbing this on a handkerchief before reaching for the painkillers.

28 soothing away eyestrain

Many headaches are caused by eyestrain. Watching a lot of television, working in poor light, long-distance driving or sitting for long periods in front of a computer screen can trigger headaches.

If your eyes are feeling tired and ache and you feel a headache coming on, you can give them a treat by covering them with cucumber slices. Or, if you are at work, you could try splashing cold water on to your eyes for a similar effect.

Alternatively, make eye-packs out of chamomile tea bags. Chamomile has a very gentle, anti-inflammatory, calming action. It helps alleviate sore, tired eyes and headaches arising from tension and anxiety. Boil a kettle and pour the hot water on to two tea bags. Leave to infuse for 10 minutes, then take them out of the water. Let them cool down and squeeze out any excess water. Lie back and place the bags over your eyes for a soothing effect.

COMPUTER USERS
If you use a computer, there are some simple steps you can take to reduce the likelihood of getting headaches from eyestrain:
• Take a short break away from your desk every 20–30 minutes.
• Make sure the computer has a good quality display and is fitted with an anti-glare filter. Adjust the brightness level on the screen to suit you.
• Set the computer screen at eye-level and position it so that it does not reflect glare from any other source of light, such as a window behind you, for instance.

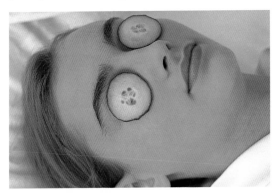

◀ Cucumber has a cooling, refreshing effect and helps to increase the circulation to the eye area.

29 feverfew

This bitter, edible plant has long been recognized as one of the most effective natural treatments for headaches and migraine. Feverfew works best as a prophylactic, taken over a period of time.

migraine cure

Science attributes the action of feverfew to a natural chemical which seems to inhibit the release of the hormone serotonin, which is thought to be a migraine trigger. A three-month course of feverfew can reduce the number and severity of attacks.

Feverfew can be taken in tablet form. Check the label and make sure the pills contain at least 0.2 per cent of the active ingredient, parthenolide. A daily dose of 200mg is usually sufficient. Alternatively, many headache and migraine sufferers have been helped by eating the fresh leaves. Eat two to three leaves daily in a brown bread sandwich. The bread makes the bitter leaves more palatable. You may also use a little honey to sweeten them.

CAUTION
- Avoid feverfew during pregnancy and while breastfeeding.
- Too much fresh feverfew can cause side effects, including mouth ulcers, stomach pain and swollen lips.
- If you are taking other medication, discuss with your doctor first.

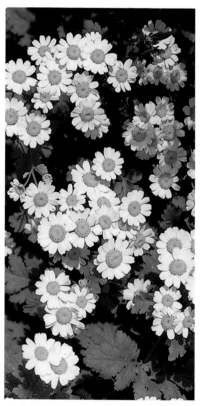

▲ Feverfew is easy to grow and can be used fresh or dried to treat headaches and migraine. The dried plant is also used to make feverfew tablets, available in good pharmacies and health stores.

30 evening primrose

For many women, headaches are a recognized symptom of PMS and of the menopause, and some women notice more headaches when taking the pill or hormone replacement therapy.

hormonal regulator

Evening primrose is a traditional North American Indian medicine and enjoys a reputation as one of nature's most valuable and versatile remedies. A great deal of research has been done on the medicinal effect of the oil, which is extracted from the plants' seeds. It is a good source of Omega-6 fatty acids, vital for the healthy functioning of the immune, nervous and hormonal systems. In particular, the oil contains gamma-linoleic acid (GLA), which is especially helpful to counter hormonal problems.

Increasingly, many women regularly take a supplement of evening primrose oil, which is available in capsule form in pharmacies and health stores. The oil is not only helpful for treating PMS, but can also assist with migraine and menopausal problems. Medicinal doses range from 500–1,500mg per day; however, for advice on dosage, talk to a healthcare professional.

◀ *The evening primrose plant is famed for its fragrant yellow flowers.*

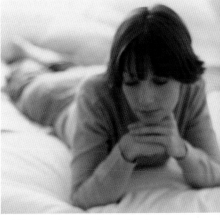

▲ *Women who suffer from migraine are most likely to suffer attacks around the time of their periods.*

HANGOVER CURE
Evening primrose oil has also been shown to counter the effects of alcoholic poisoning. For a hangover headache, try taking a couple of capsules instead of a painkiller.

CAUTION
Evening primrose should be avoided by women with breast cancer and sufferers of epilepsy.

31 herbal steam inhalant

A stuffy nose and blocked sinuses can sometimes be the cause of a headache. Steam inhalations are a good way of clearing the head. The addition of fresh herbs will help to relieve the headache.

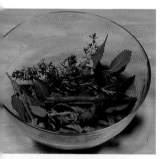

1 To clear the sinuses and ease a congestive headache, gather together a large handful of lavender, rosemary, peppermint, sage, thyme and eucalyptus. Put the selected herbs in a bowl.

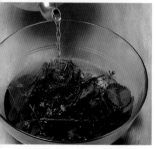

2 Pour on 1 litre/ 1¾ pints/4 cups of boiling water. Lavender and rosemary are natural painkillers, while peppermint and eucalyptus are good for clearing blocked noses and throats.

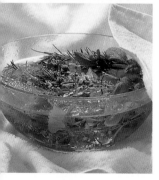

3 Lean over the bowl, with a towel draped over your head and shoulders to form a tent. Breathe in the steamy vapour as deeply as possible. The inhalation will decongest blocked nasal passages, kill any germs and clear the headache.

TIPS
• If fresh herbs are not available, then an inhalation using essential oils of peppermint, eucalyptus, lavender and rosemary may be tried instead. Use 2 drops of each oil to 1 litre/1¾ pints/4 cups of boiling water.

• The hormonal action of thyme can help lift depression and the symptoms of fatigue.

CAUTION
If you have high blood pressure or asthma, seek medical advice before using steam inhalants. Eucalyptus and peppermint may interfere with homeopathic remedies.

32 comforting compress

Many headache sufferers find a compress helps their symptoms. A compress is a cloth which has been soaked in water with a few drops of essential oil added, wrung out, then applied to the head.

Of all the essential oils used in the treatment of headaches, lavender and peppermint seem to be the most effective. Although they can be used separately, these oils work well together. Both are painkillers and complement each other: lavender is a sedative while peppermint is a stimulant. This dual action is found in many commercial headache remedies, which include a stimulant (such as caffeine) to counteract the slightly sedative, and even depressing effect of the painkiller. The important difference is that essential oils do not just suppress the pain but get to work on the cause of the headache. A compress will be most effective if it is used immediately at the onset of a headache.

you will need
600ml/1 pint/2½ cups
   cold water
bowl
2–3 drops lavender
   essential oil
2–3 drops peppermint
   essential oil
piece of soft cotton
   fabric

1 Pour the water into the bowl. When the water is still add the essential oils and gently stir the water to disperse the oils.
2 Fold the soft cotton fabric into a loose pad. Place it on the surface of the water and let it soak up the essential oils. Wring it out lightly.
3 Place the compress across the forehead to relieve the headache. As soon as it gets warm, soak it again in the water and re-apply.

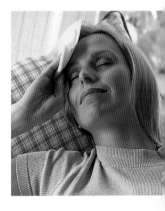

TIPS
- During a migraine attack, some sufferers cannot tolerate the smell of peppermint, in which case try alternating hot and cold lavender compresses.
- A cold compress on the back of the neck will ease a tension headache, and one on the forehead is best for a thumping headache.

33

lime blossom tisane

A simple but effective way of curing a headache is to drink a herbal tea. Lime blossom and lemon balm (*Melissa*) leaves make a delicately fragranced drink for soothing tension headaches.

herbal infusions

Making herbal tisanes from fresh ingredients increases their potency and medicinal value. Lime flowers have a relaxing and cleansing effect in the body. They can help with high blood pressure, and are effective in treating headaches, including migraine. Lime flowers make a good remedy for any condition associated with tension, including depression, and back, neck and shoulder pain. Lemon balm is useful for calming tension and promoting feelings of well-being; it also relieves headaches and migraine. The two herbs are complementary.

To make this tisane, gather a handful each of lemon balm leaves and lime blossom – pick lime blossom when the flowers are just opening. Use five or six fresh flowers and leaves per cup, and drop them into near-boiling water. Cover and leave to steep for three or four minutes. Strain off the liquid and drink hot or cold, three times a day. The tea has a fresh, lemony taste.

◀ *Lime blossom can also be mixed with peppermint for a more uplifting effect.*

CAUTION
Although natural, herbal teas can be potent and should be taken no more than three times a day and for no more than two weeks at a time.

34 wood betony infusion

Once considered a panacea for all ills, wood betony may be used alone or combined with lavender or rosemary to make a soothing herbal infusion to ease your headache.

The leaves and pink flowering tops of wood betony are used in medicinal preparations. The plant has a stimulating effect on the circulation and is also a relaxant, making it helpful for both congestive and tension headaches. It is also a tonic to the nervous system, helping to ease anxiety, lift depression and soothe pain.

The infusion may be made with either fresh or dried ingredients. Fill a cup with near-boiling water and add 5ml/1 tsp dried wood betony and 2.5ml/½ tsp dried lavender or rosemary. Double these quantities if you are using fresh herbs. Cover and leave to steep for 10 minutes. Strain and drink, sweetened with a little honey if required.

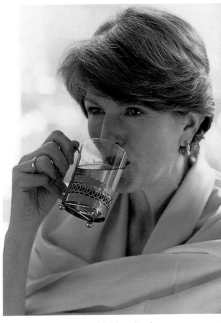

▲ Wood betony was highly prized as a medicinal herb in Roman times. The Anglo-Saxons believed it capable of driving away despair.

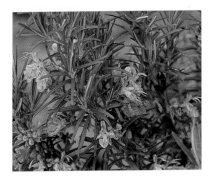

◄ Fresh rosemary is invigorating and refreshing. It is excellent for clearing congestive headaches, and combines well with wood betony to relieve nervous tension.

35 herbal sedatives

Headaches caused by stress and nervous exhaustion are generally linked with an inability to switch the mind off and relax, leading to insomnia and restless nights.

calming the nerves

There are several herbs which have a strong sedative action and which are useful for headaches associated with nervous exhaustion and overactivity. Among the most commonly used are valerian, vervain and sweet marjoram: any one of these can be made into an infusion that will help you to relax and promote restful, healing sleep. Do not take all three together.

For every 250ml/8fl oz/1 cup of near-boiling water you will need 10ml/2 tsp of fresh valerian, vervain or sweet marjoram. If using dried herbs, halve the quantity. Drop the herbs into the water, cover and leave to infuse for 5–10 minutes. Strain off the liquid, sweeten with a little honey, and drink before going to bed.

> **CAUTION**
> Sweet marjoram and vervain should not be taken during pregnancy. Valerian should not be taken by anyone with liver disease.

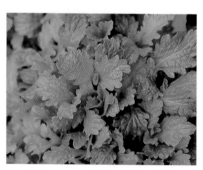

▲ Vervain is a wonderful tonic for the nervous system, calming the nerves and easing tension. It protects against stress, and is useful for treating headaches caused by anxiety, depression and insomnia.

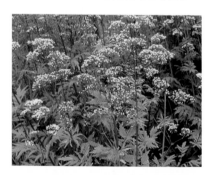

▲ Valerian has a calming effect on the mind and helps to relax tense muscles – use it to ease a tight neck and shoulders. It is a strong sedative, and forms the basis of the pharmaceutical drug, valium.

36 lavender tincture

Tinctures are an effective way to extract the active ingredients of plants. They are made with fresh or dried herbs which are steeped in a mixture of alcohol and water. This one will cure a headache.

you will need
15g/½oz dried lavender
250ml/8fl oz/1 cup vodka, made
  up to 300ml/½ pint/1¼ cups
  with water
dark glass jar with an airtight lid

1 Put the dried lavender into a glass jar and pour in the vodka and water mixture. It will almost immediately start to turn a beautiful lavender blue.
2 Put a lid on the jar and leave in a cool, dark place for 7–10 days (no longer), shaking the jar occasionally. The tincture will eventually turn dark purple.
3 Strain off the lavender through a sieve lined with a paper towel before pouring into a sterilized glass bottle. Seal with a tight-fitting lid and store in a cool, dark place for future use.

As tinctures are highly concentrated medicinal extracts, take no more than 5ml/1 tsp, three or four times a day, as a headache treatment. The tincture may be diluted in a little water or fruit juice. Alternatively, a few drops may be added to a compress.

MEDICINE CHEST
• Among herbal remedies, tinctures have a relatively long shelf-life; properly stored, they will keep for up to two years, as the alcohol acts as a preservative.
• Lavender tincture is a useful remedy to have on standby as it can be used to treat many common health problems, such as burns, muscular aches and pains, coughs and colds, as well as headaches of all kinds.

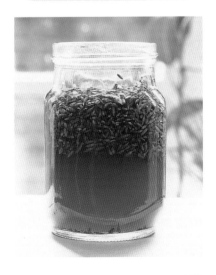

37   replenish the system

Many headaches, including those caused by a hangover, are the direct result of dehydration or low blood sugar. There are several simple remedies to counteract or avoid such problems altogether.

rehydrate

To keep the body fully hydrated, it's important to drink plenty of water – aim for at least 2 litres/3½ pints a day – and to avoid drinking too many diuretic drinks such as tea, coffee, cola and alcohol. Help to stay hydrated by eating food with a high water content and make your own fruit and vegetable juices. Drink a glass of water as soon as you get up and at least half-an-hour before each meal. Sip water at 10–15 minute intervals during exercise. Be sure to drink a glass of water at the first sign of a headache.

Vitamin C

Vitamin C is needed for more than 300 metabolic processes in the body. Kiwi fruit and all citrus fruits are a good natural source. Make a drink from freshly squeezed orange or lemon juice, sweeten it with honey and it will help your headache.

fruit sugar

Hangover headaches seem to result from alcohol-induced disturbances in the brain. This may cause low blood sugar, which is why eating a high

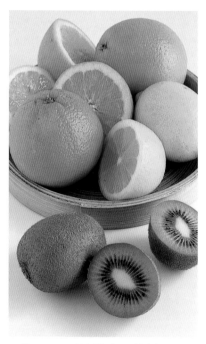

▲ *Oranges and kiwi fruit are high in vitamin C.*

fructose (fruit sugar) snack before going to bed may help. It is thought that fructose helps metabolize the chemical products. Fructose is found in carrots, and in all fruits, especially dates. Fructose bars are also available.

38

Bach flower remedies

The Bach flower remedies work on any underlying emotional or psychological cause of a headache, treating the negative mental and emotional states which lead to pain and tension in the body.

Dr Edward Bach discovered the healing energies of selected flowering plants and trees, by "tuning in" to their subtle vibrations. He noted that the plants affected him on a mental and emotional level, and devised a system of healing based on these states. The remedies match certain personality types and are chosen accordingly.

Bach flower essences are gentle and safe to use and are available in most pharmacies and health stores. They may be taken separately or in a combination of up to six remedies. They may also be taken in conjunction with other treatments. Add a couple of drops of each essence to a glass of water and sip at frequent intervals.

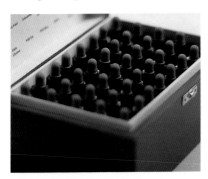
▲ There are 38 Bach essences.

FLOWER ESSENCES

To treat a headache, select from the following remedies:

- **Beech** if you are critical and intolerant of others and yourself.
- **Cherry Plum** if you have repressed anger and feel as if you might explode, or feel fearful.
- **Crab Apple** if you try to be "superman/woman", or are driven by the need to be perfect.
- **Gorse** if you have feelings of hopelessness and are resigned to fate.
- **Holly** if you suffer from feelings of jealousy, hatred, resentment and frustration.
- **Impatiens** if you feel tension due to rapid mental activity, or are always in a hurry.
- **Pine** if you have feelings of guilt and inferiority, if you always blame yourself or are always apologizing.
- **Vervain** if you live on your nerves, are keyed up and unable to relax.
- **Vine** if you are rigid in your thinking, if you are inflexible or ambitious, or if you think you are always right.
- **White Chestnut** for thoughts that go round and round.

massage with oils

Gentle massage of the temples and forehead can help to stop a tension headache from getting a tight grip and encourage the body to relax. Use essential oils for additional benefit.

Everyone can benefit from the comforting touch of massage. The sense of touch is a powerful tool of communication and can be used to benefit the recipient on an emotional, physical and mental level. It helps relaxation, relieves aching muscles and reduces pain making it a useful treatment for headaches.

Add any of the essential oils in the quantity stated in the box, right, to 30ml/2 tbsp of a light vegetable oil, such as almond or grapeseed, or to an unscented cream or lotion.

CHOOSING AN OIL
• **Rosemary** for a congestive headache. Rosemary is uplifting and clears the mind. Use 4 drops.
• **Peppermint** if the head feels too hot (peppermint has a cooling action). Use 4 drops.
• **Lavender** if warmth feels as though it is helpful. Use 6 drops.
• **Chamomile** for either headaches or migraine. Use 4 drops.
• **Marjoram** when the mind simply won't switch off. Use 4 drops.

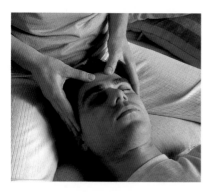

1 With your thumbs, use steady but gentle pressure to stroke the forehead and work the oils into the skin. The strokes will help ease tension.

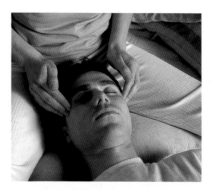

2 Gently massage the temples with the tips of your fingers to release tension and stress. Work the oils into the skin as before.

40 neck & shoulder easer

Sitting hunched over a desk for long periods, driving, or carrying heavy bags are just a few of the occupational hazards that create tension in the shoulders, neck and below the ridge of the skull.

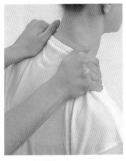

1 Anchor your fingers over the shoulders. Roll and squeeze the muscles in a kneading action, working out to the edge of the shoulders and down the tops of the arms.

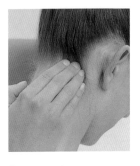

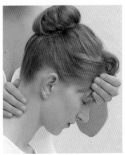

2 Place one hand across the forehead and the other across the nape of the neck. Squeeze the muscles of the neck between the fingers and heel of your hand.

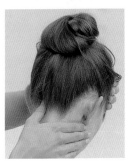

3 Supporting the forehead, use the thumb pad of the other hand to press upwards into the hollow at the top of the spine below the skull. Apply gentle upward pressure for a steady count of five, then release.

4 Loosen the constricted muscles under the base of the skull by massaging beneath the bony ridge, working from the top of the spine to the outer edge of the skull.

5 Change hands to massage beneath the other side of the skull. Ease scalp tension by rotating the fingertips of both hands in small circles all over the head.

41 shoulder reliever

Having a shoulder massage is one of the best ways of releasing muscular tension. It not only feels good, but can help to prevent or ease a headache. Practise this routine with a friend or your partner.

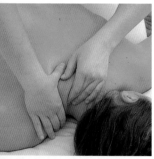

1 Make sure your partner faces away from you. Place both your hands on one shoulder, and with alternate hands squeeze your fingers and thumb together. Repeat on the other side.

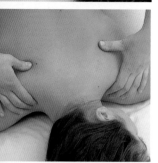

2 Place your thumbs on each side of the spine on the upper back, with the rest of each hand over each shoulder. Squeeze your fingers and thumbs together, rolling the flesh between them.

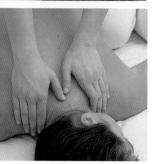

3 Let your thumbs smoothly move out across the shoulder muscles, and release the pressure of the thumbs as you stretch the shoulder blades outwards, away from the spine, with your hands.

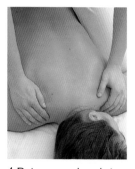

4 Return your hands to the centre and repeat this movement with a firm kneading action.

RELAX
A typical response to feeling burdened by life's responsibilities is to tighten up in the trapezius, the large muscle in our shoulders. We hold a lot of tension in this area; when you feel "uptight" it is often the shoulders that bear the load. Make a conscious effort to relax your shoulders.

42 anxiety calmer

When you are feeling anxious and upset, the muscles of the face tense up, making you look fraught. Having the face gently massaged is very relaxing, and a great way to soothe a headache.

Ask a friend to practise this routine with you. It is best done when you have an opportunity to relax afterwards. For a headache, it is a good idea to use essential oils, blended in a little massage oil. Choose a light vegetable oil, such as sweet almond or grapeseed, as a base. Use four or five drops of essential oil to 30ml/ 2 tbsp massage oil, but take care not to put too much on at a time, as most people don't like a greasy feeling on the face. If you prefer, you may use an unscented lotion or cream as a base.

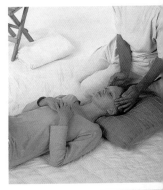

1 Ideally have the person lying down with the head on a cushion. With your fingertips, smooth the essential oil blend into the face. Pay particular attention to the temples and forehead, using small circular movements and light brushing strokes.

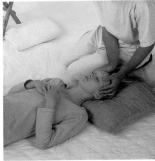

2 Using your thumbs one after the other, stroke tension away from the centre of the forehead. Finish the routine by holding your hands still on each side of the face; this feels very calming and reassuring.

ESSENTIAL OILS
• **Chamomile** or **marjoram** for headaches that are the result of overwork, anger or worry.
• **Lavender** for migraine and tension headaches.
• **Tea tree** for clearing the head.

43 shiatsu massage

This Japanese healing system applies gentle pressure to the body using stretching and holding movements. Tension headaches can be eased by focusing on the neck, shoulder and temple areas.

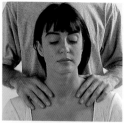

1 Standing behind your partner, place both hands loosely on each side of the neck. Gently massage the shoulders to help relax your partner's breathing.

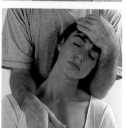

2 Tilt the head sideways and support with your hand. Place the forearm across the shoulder and apply downward pressure. Repeat on the other side.

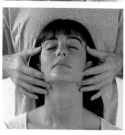

3 Apply gentle pressure with the thumb and forefinger from the base of the neck to the nape. Hold at the nape for 5 seconds, then release. Next, tilt the head back, supporting it. Place your thumbs on the temples with the fingers resting on each side of the face. Rotate the thumbs using a small circular motion, in a clockwise direction.

POSTURE
Sit on an upright chair with good back support.

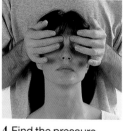

4 Find the pressure points just above the inner corner of each eye. Apply gentle pressure with the middle fingers to help disperse the pain. Hold for 5 seconds.

5 Position your thumbs about 5cm/2in apart on each side of the head, just above the hairline, with the palms pressed flat along the sides of the face. Press the thumbs evenly back along the top of the head.

facial massage

Because of the very high number of nerve receptors on the facial skin's surface, face massage is a mainline to relaxation. It not only helps the muscles let off tension, but also sends relaxing signals to the brain.

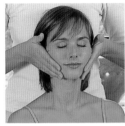

1 Standing behind your partner, softly draw your hands down the face, following the jawline, to cup the face at the base of the jaw. Then slowly draw your fingers and palms up over the face, trailing them across the cheeks and up to the tops of the ears. Extend this stroke to sweep over the eye sockets and take in the forehead. Repeat this final movement a few times to encourage the facial muscles to relax.

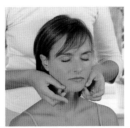

2 Return your hands to cup the bottom of the face and place your thumb and index finger of each at the centre of the chin. With your thumbs on top and index fingers underneath, gently pick up the fold of flesh along the chin and roll it between your fingers. Work along just under the edge of the jaw line towards the ears. Repeat three times.

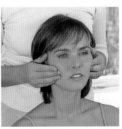

3 At the jaw sockets, make circular strokes with your fingertips as shown, with particular attention to the hinge area. If your partner is holding their jaw tight, you could ask them to drop their mouth open to help release tension.

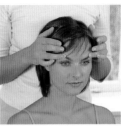

4 Use your fingers to gently press at three evenly spaced points along the eyebrow. Begin at the inner edge of the brow and finish at the outer. Repeat the stroke directly above these points in the middle of the forehead, and lastly at the very top of the forehead. Repeat the seqence a further two times. Finish this sequence by stroking the forehead.

CAUTION
You can give or receive Shiatsu as often as you wish, but there are times when it is not appropriate. Avoid treating a partner who:
• has a high fever
• is intoxicated
• is suffering from high blood pressure
• is in the first three months of pregnancy
• is suffering from a contagious disease or blood-borne cancer

44 reflexology

The science of reflexology believes that our bodies are reflected in miniature in our feet. If we treat the specific area of the foot that represents the head, we can massage away a headache.

an ancient art

Having a reflexology treatment is relaxing and can treat specific health problems. It is effective for treating tension headaches as well as for migraines.

Your head is represented on the toes; the right side of your head lies on the right big toe and the left side on the left big toe. In addition, the eight other toes contain the reflexes to specific parts of your head, for fine tuning. By applying gentle pressure to these exact points, reflexology stimulates the body to heal itself.

Reflexology can be an excellent preventive therapy. If the headache is a symptom of another illness, a different part of the foot to that suggested here would need to be treated first.

1 Work the hypothalmus reflex first, as this controls the release of endorphins for the relief of pain.

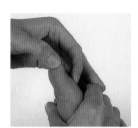

2 Work down the spine to take pressure away from the head. This will draw energy down the body and ground it.

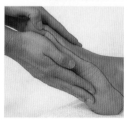

3 Work the cervical spine on the big toe. Work the neck of all the toes to relieve tension.

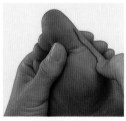

4 Work the diaphragm to encourage freer breathing. Repeat the reflexology treatment on the other foot.

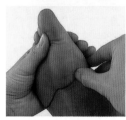

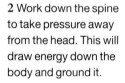

45   scalp massage

A scalp massage is deeply relaxing. If you are suffering from stress-related headaches, use this treatment on a regular basis to reduce tension. It only takes a few minutes.

If you are stressed, the scalp muscles tighten. One side effect is that the roots of your hair become starved of nourishment and your hair will start to thin out and weaken. This massage stimulates the hair roots. The advantage of this massage is that it is one you can do for yourself.

▶ *Lank, lifeless hair is often a sign of stress.*

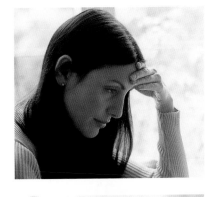

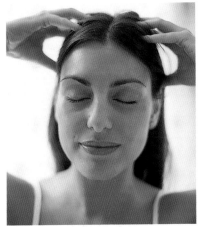

1 Place the thumbs at the top of the ears and "glue" the fingers to the scalp, moving it firmly and slowly over the bone beneath.

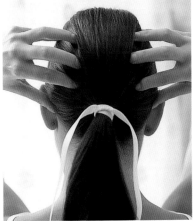

2 Place the hands on another part of the scalp and repeat. Carry on until the whole scalp has been covered. Repeat steps 1 and 2 several times.

46 head revitalizer

This simple self-massage sequence will help to ease headaches, whatever their cause. You can also use it to increase your vitality and help you to focus your mind throughout the day.

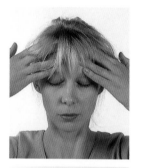

1 Use small, circling movements with the fingers, working steadily from the forehead down around the temples and over the cheeks.

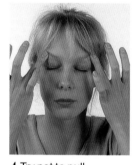

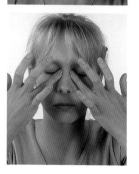

2 Use firm pressure and work slowly to ease tensions out of all the facial muscles. Use your fingers to gently press around the eye sockets, by the nose.

3 Smooth firmly around the arcs of the eye sockets. Work across the cheeks and along each side of the nose, then move out to the jaw line where a lot of tension is held.

4 Try not to pull downwards on the skin – let the circling movements help to smooth the stresses away and gently lift the face as you work.

USE AN OIL
If you are feeling overwrought, make up an aromatherapy blend of 4 drops lavender and 2 drops ylang ylang in 30ml/ 2 tbsp of a light massage oil, such as sweet almond or grapeseed.

47 migraine easers

Having a migraine is one of nature's ways of shutting the body down when things get too much. Rather than trying to "fight it off", respect what your body is saying and look after yourself.

There are several essential oils which can help a migraine, but use them sparingly and carefully. Many migraine sufferers have a heightened sense of smell at the onset of an attack, and may find any aroma intolerable.

Alternatively, use a drop of each oil in a bowl of warm water, and apply a warm compress to the forehead. If this blend smells too strong, you could just try lavender on its own, 3–4 drops in the base oil or cream as before.

massage mix

As soon as you feel a migraine coming on, try a massage blend of 2 drops rosemary, 1 drop marjoram, and 1 drop clary sage oil, diluted in 30ml/2 tbsp of a light vegetable oil, such as grapeseed or sweet almond. You may use an unscented lotion or cream base rather than oil if you prefer.

1 Using the massage mix, gently rub the temples with small circular movements, using the tips of your fingers.

2 If touching the head does not make the pain worse, ask a friend to give you a gentle head massage. This can feel very soothing and comforting and help you to relax.

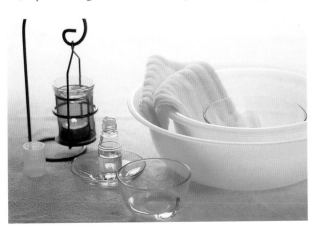

◄ *Migraine headaches are not the same as everyday tension headaches, and if you suffer from these you should seek professional advice.*

48 calming sleep massage

The gentle wave-like strokes of this massage wash over and down the body and legs with a deliciously hypnotic and sedative effect – ideal to ease away headaches before going to sleep.

1 Place one hand over the chest and the other over the back of the shoulder. As you breathe in, pull your hands steadily outwards and down to the edge of the shoulder. Pause briefly as you exhale, lightly cradling the top of the arm.

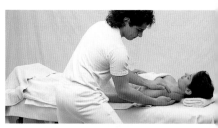

2 Continue the pulling motion down the length of the arm. As you breathe in, pull both hands down to just below the elbow joint. Relax as you breathe out, then continue the slide down the forearm and below the wrist.

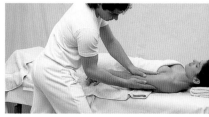

3 Draw your hands over both sides of your partner's hand and fingers, taking your stroke out beyond the body as the hand settles back on to the mattress. Repeat steps 1–3 on the other side of the body.

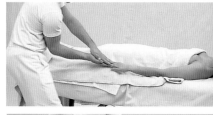

4 Pull your hands down over the hips and down the leg to just below the knee. Continue this wave-like motion down the lower leg to the ankle, then pull gently and steadily out over the toes. Repeat this sequence of strokes on the other side of the body. Repeat each movement up to five times.

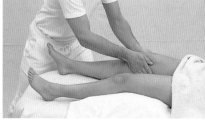

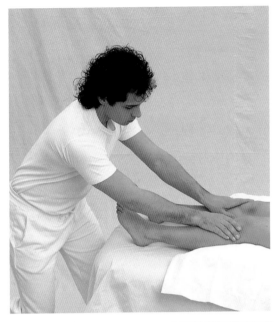

5 Using the flat surface of both hands, softly stroke down the legs from the thighs until your hands pass over and out of the feet. Repeat the movement as many times as you like to allow your partner to relax.

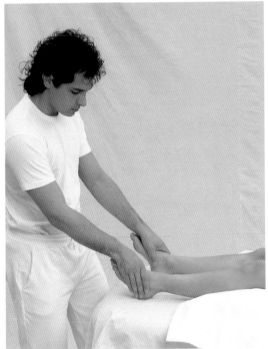

6 To increase the sedative effect of your strokes, complete these sequences with a still, calm hold of your hands over the front of both feet. This will draw the energy down the body, bringing a sense of balance and peace to the recipient.

49 draw out the pain

Certain techniques can help to release the pain of a tension headache. Those shown here all involve applying pressure then releasing it. This helps to relax the muscles and draw the pain away.

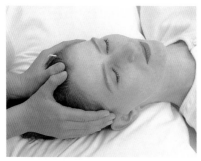

1 Settle your hands lightly around your partner's scalp for a few moments. Keeping your hands in the cupped position, lift them slowly away from the head as if they are drawing out the pain. Cup your hands around the head again, placing your thumbs between the eyebrows. Apply gentle pressure with your thumbs for a count of five, then release.

2 Working from inner to outer edge, apply a press/release motion under the ridge of both eyebrows using the tips of your index fingers. Then use your thumb pads to press/release over the top of the cheekbones, working out from the nose to the edge of the temples.

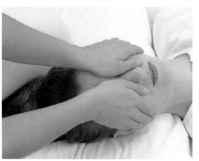

3 Briskly rub your hands together to create heat, then softly lay your slightly cupped palms over the eyes for a count of five to soothe and relax the eye muscles. Withdraw your hands slowly.

50 tension reliever

Tension headaches are a common consequence of stressful lifestyles. This massage can prevent muscle spasm and head pain, particularly if it is done at the onset of a headache.

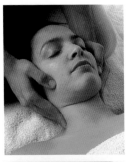

1 Kneel at your partner's head with the head in your lap or on a cushion. Begin by making circles with your fingertips on the muscles at each side of the neck. Continue around the sides of the head and behind the ears.

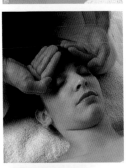

2 Use the backs of your hands to smooth tension away from the temples. Gently stroke the hands outwards across the forehead to soothe away worry lines.

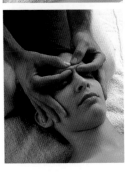

3 Pinch and gently squeeze along the line of the eyebrows, reducing pressure as you work outwards. These muscles may be very tender, so take care.

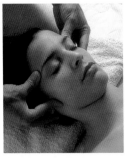

4 With your thumbs, use steady but firm pressure on the forehead, working outwards from between the eyebrows.

5 Work across the brow to the hair line. This also covers many acupressure points, and will release blocked energy.

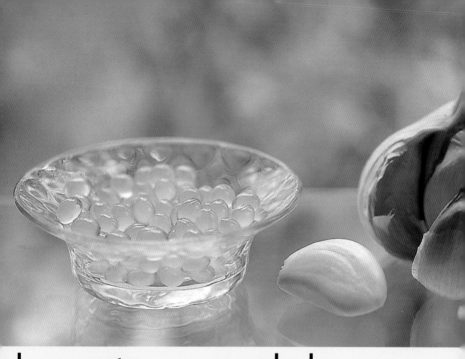

beat a cold

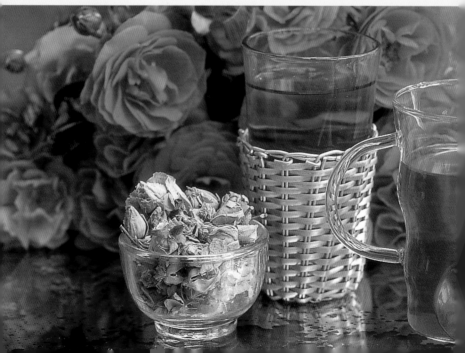

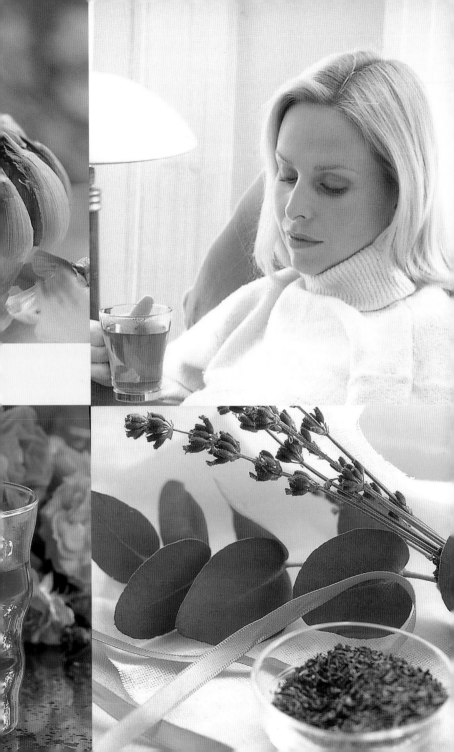

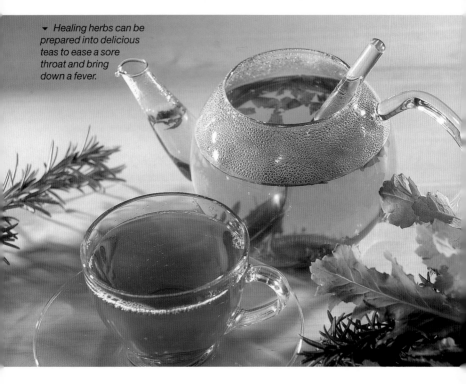

▼ Healing herbs can be prepared into delicious teas to ease a sore throat and bring down a fever.

how to get rid of a cold

A cold is reputedly the most common infection that you are likely to suffer. With over 200 strains of cold virus and new flu-strains cropping up every winter, huge numbers of the population can expect to "go down" with a cold or flu-like symptoms at least once or twice a year.

With so many different cold viruses, it is perhaps not surprising that a miracle cure has not been found. Instead, a plethora of over-the-counter preparations exist to help you cope with the unpleasant symptoms of colds and flu. Generally, these treatments are based on suppressing the body's symptoms,

"knocking them on the head" so that you can carry on with your life as normal. One of the problems with many pharmaceutical drug-based products however, is that they often have undesirable side effects, which can create a new set of problems for the body. In the long term, they may even have a weakening effect on the immune system as it copes with the toxic residue from chemically produced compounds. This has encouraged a growing interest in traditional natural remedies, safely practised for hundreds of years, as people look for effective treatments that are gentle and non-toxic.

what is a cold?

The common cold is a viral infection affecting the upper respiratory system: the nose, throat and sinus passages. Every day, the air that you breathe contains many harmful viruses (pathogens), which the respiratory tract works hard to combat, fighting them off before they enter the body.

One of the body's first lines of defence is the nose: you rely on it to trap and neutralize pathogens. With central heating and a lack of fresh air, the mucus membranes of the nose and sinuses become swollen and congested with a thick secretion. When the respiratory system cannot deal with the pathogens effectively, they enter the body tissue where they begin to damage cells, causing inflammation and all the other cold-like symptoms.

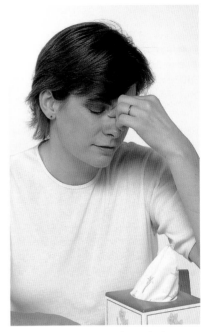

▲ A blocked-up nose is the perfect breeding ground for germs.

general symptoms

Colds usually come on suddenly and the symptoms are relatively mild and of limited duration, lasting on average a week to ten days. Typically, the first stage of a cold is characterized by sneezing, watery eyes and a sore throat as the mucus membranes become inflamed. This may be accompanied by shivering and feeling chilly, usually a sign of a raised temperature as the body attempts to kill off the invading germs. Other signs of a raised temperature include aching limbs and feeling weak, as the viruses spread beyond the primary site of infection (in the nose and throat), into the blood and on to different organs and tissues in the body. The body then becomes vulnerable to secondary respiratory infections such as sinusitis, laryngitis, ear infections and bronchitis, which are usually more unpleasant and much more serious than the original cold.

During a cold the body produces more mucus in order to help trap the invading germs. Once the drippy, runny nose stage dries up, it can turn into a blocked, stuffed-up head cold, which may also be accompanied by a cough.

coughs

A cough is a reflex action of the bronchi, designed to clear the airways of excessive mucus. Coughs can be divided into two types, each needing different treatments. A loose, moist "productive" cough needs remedies that help the body to expel the excess mucus. With a dry, tickling cough, the mucus membranes have become so inflamed that they provoke coughing even when there is no mucus to clear. This type of cough can be exhausting and calls for treatments that soothe the inflammation and help to reduce aggravating bronchial spasm.

catching a cold

The common-sense belief is that colds are created through catching a germ. Although this statement is partly true, it doesn't explain why some people catch colds and others, even if they have been exposed to the same virus, do not. First, you have to create a suitable breeding ground in the body before a germ can take hold. When you catch a cold, it means that your immune system is below par in some way and your body is unable to fight off infection. There are various reasons why this may be so, and there are many things that you can do to try to prevent this happening.

lifestyle indicators

Research indicates that many respiratory problems originate in an unhealthy lifestyle. Lack of fresh air and exercise, shallow breathing, poor posture, smoking and air pollution all place a strain on the lungs. Similarly, eating a diet high in dairy produce, sugar and refined carbohydrates places a strain on the body, as these foods weaken the immune system

and encourage the build-up of mucus. Good health is linked with a balanced lifestyle. Regular exercise, sufficient rest and sleep, a balanced diet, satisfying work and fulfilling relationships all contribute towards health and well-being.

When any area of life is out of balance, it places a strain on the immune system. The greater the duration and level of stress, the more the immune system is weakened. You can encourage the immune system to stay strong and healthy by drinking more fresh juices and mineral water, and eating plenty of organic fruit, vegetables and salad.

holistic medicine

In natural medicine, a cold is not necessarily seen as a bad thing as it may be the body's way of trying to clear out toxins from the system and of giving the body a much-needed rest. Consequently, natural treatments are not based on ignoring and/or suppressing a cold, but are designed to work with the body, recognizing its symptoms as part of the body's self-healing process.

Holistic medicine is about finding ways to encourage your body to stay strong and healthy, and using drug-free treatments, free from side effects, whenever you do become sick.

Whether you are suffering from a runny nose, a sore throat, aching limbs, a raised temperature or blocked sinuses, this section is packed with a variety of non-pharmaceutical remedies to help alleviate your symptoms.

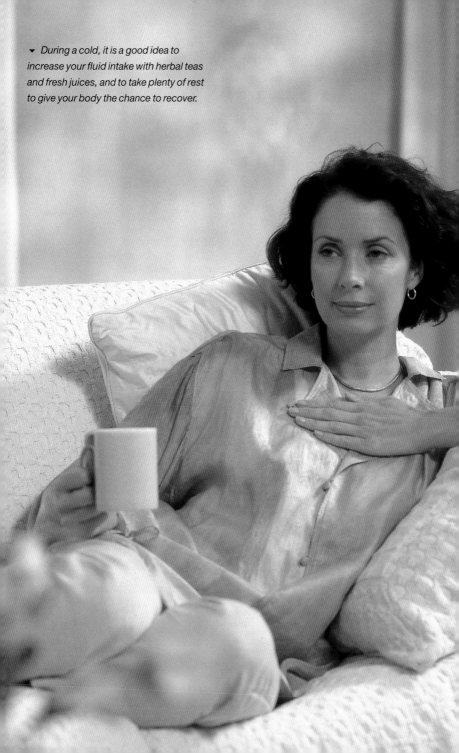

▼ *During a cold, it is a good idea to increase your fluid intake with herbal teas and fresh juices, and to take plenty of rest to give your body the chance to recover.*

cold treatments

There are literally hundreds of natural remedies
that can heal and soothe a cold and strengthen
the immune system. The following pages contain
50 of the most effective methods, many of which
have been tried and tested for centuries and used
in different healing traditions across the world.
All the treatments are based on holistic principles
– where the pathway to health is seen as a fine
balance between mental, physical and emotional
wellbeing – and are designed to stimulate the
body's own healing ability. They include energy
therapies, such as homeopathy, reiki and crystal
healing, as well as hands-on methods, such
as massage and reflexology. There are also
treatments based on nutrition, vitamins, minerals
and medicinal foods, together with many herbal
remedies, utilizing a plant's leaves, fruits and
flowers to make gargles, teas, cordials, syrups,
lotions and tonics. With 50 natural treatments to
choose from, you're bound to find the remedy
to suit your needs.

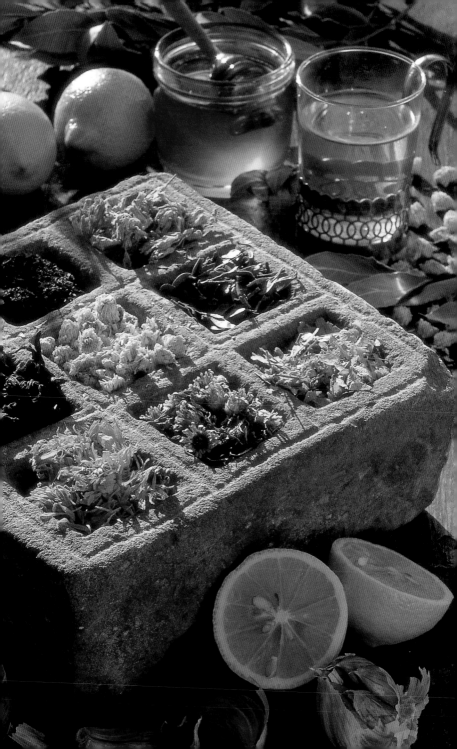

51 strengthening vitamin C

A strong immune system is vital for good health. Vitamin C plays an essential role in supporting the immune system to fight infection, and has potent antiviral and antibacterial properties.

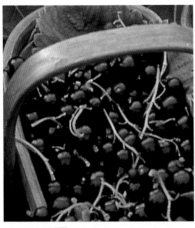

▲ Fresh blackcurrants are a good source of vitamin C. Eat them lightly cooked or raw.

Vitamin C is used up more rapidly under stress and when fighting colds or infection. The body is unable to store or produce this water-soluble vitamin, and relies on an adequate daily intake. For this reason, vitamin C is generally regarded as safe to take in therapeutic doses, as any excess is excreted via the kidneys.

For treating colds, many health care practitioners recommend a therapeutic dose of 1000mg taken three times a day. This should be gradually reduced to one 1000mg dose taken once a day, then to 500mg a day as a maintenance dose to keep coughs and colds at bay. Therapeutic doses of vitamin C are best taken as a dietary supplement in the form of tablets or effervescent powders.

The best natural sources of vitamin C are fruit and vegetables, particularly citrus fruits, blackcurrants, berries, rosehips, (bell) peppers, green leafy vegetables, carrots and sweet potatoes. It is best to consume these foods raw (except for rosehips and potatoes), as vitamin C is destroyed by cooking.

BEST FOOD SOURCES OF VITAMIN C IN MG PER 100G

Rosehip syrup	295
Blackcurrants	200
Guavas	200
Parsley	150
Broccoli	110
Green peppers	100
Citrus fruits	50–80
Watercress	60
All other fruit and vegetables	20–40

52 essential zinc

Lowered zinc levels impair the healthy functioning of the immune system. If you feel run down, suffer frequent colds and have a poor sense of taste or smell, it could be that you are deficient in zinc.

Zinc is an essential mineral that is involved in many bodily processes and is necessary for normal cell division and function. Unfortunately research indicates that zinc deficiencies are fairly common in large numbers of the population. The body's reserves of zinc are depleted by stress, vigorous exercise (the mineral is lost through excessive sweating), smoking, and high intakes of tea, coffee, alcohol and refined foods. Even if you eat plenty of fresh fruit and vegetables, they are likely to have been grown in soils that are low in vital minerals and trace elements, including zinc.

One of the best natural sources of zinc is shellfish, particularly oysters, crabs and mussels. Liver and dried brewer's yeast are also high in zinc, and other sources include hard cheese, eggs, beef, turkey and pumpkin seeds.

To make sure you are getting enough zinc, take a zinc supplement of between 15–20mg a day with a glass of orange juice (vitamin C aids zinc absorption). Zinc supplements should not be taken on an empty stomach as they may cause nausea.

For a cold, you could try sucking zinc lozenges, which are available in good health stores and pharmacies. It seems that the mineral may have a direct action on the cold viruses in the mouth, nose and throat, which stops them multiplying.

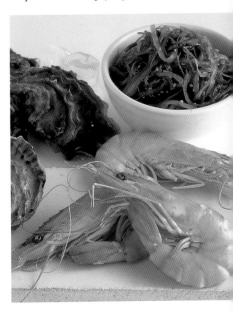

▸ *Making shellfish a regular part of your diet will help to increase your zinc levels.*

herbal infusions

People have been making simple home remedies for combating the effects of coughs and colds for thousands of years. All that is required is a teapot or small pan and the appropriate herb.

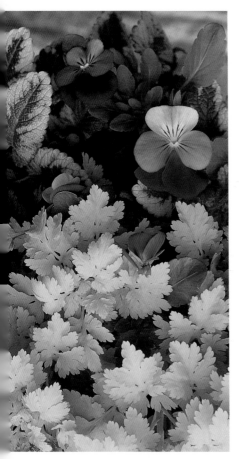

▲ *An infusion of heartsease or wild pansy is useful for treating colds and coughs.*

Many common herbs have been used over the centuries for concocting effective treatments for sneezes and wheezes. Heartsease (*Viola tricolor*) and sweet violet (*V. odorata*) teas were traditionally used for treating colds, while the reputation of horehound (*Marrubium vulgare*) goes back at least to the 1st century AD, when it was renowned as a remedy for coughs and colds. Horehound and ginger tea, using 1 teaspoon powdered ginger with the herb leaves, is an excellent cold remedy. Combined with hyssop, sage or thyme, horehound makes a soothing gargle for sore throats. It was also boiled up with sugar to make cough candy. With its reputation for lowering fever, catmint may be taken as an infusion for the relief of a feverish cold or influenza.

To make a tea or infusion put 15g/½oz roughly chopped fresh herb leaves into a pot and pour in 600ml/1 pint/2½ cups boiling water. Cover and leave to infuse for 5–7 minutes. Strain off the leaves and sweeten with honey.

54 antiseptic garlic

King of all healing plants, garlic is one of nature's "swear by" remedies. This powerful antiseptic was regularly used to treat all kinds of infections before the development of antibiotics.

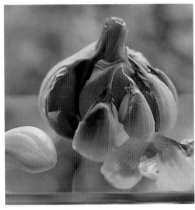

▲ *An average clove of garlic contains substances equivalent to roughly one-fifth of an average penicillin dose.*

To get the most from garlic's health-giving properties, get into the habit of adding a little to your daily diet – it will help keep you strong and healthy.

Raw garlic is best, but one of the problems with garlic is its pungent odour and taste, which is not to everyone's liking. Eating fresh parsley or tarragon helps to reduce garlic breath, and lightly stir-frying the cloves for a few moments also helps to eliminate any unpleasant after-effects. The cloves can be crushed, chopped or left whole, with crushed garlic having the strongest flavour. When cooking, make sure that the garlic does not turn brown as this will make it taste bitter. Add the garlic to food prior to serving.

To treat a cold, you should eat up to six fresh cloves a day. If you cannot bear the taste or smell, odourless garlic capsules are widely available from health food stores as well as most supermarkets. You should take 1–3 garlic capsules daily.

- Garlic has antibacterial and antiviral properties and a long tradition of medicinal use. Slaves in ancient Egypt were fed it to keep them strong, traditional Chinese herbalists prescribed it, chewed raw, to keep coughs and colds at bay, and both ancient Greek and Roman physicians prescribed garlic to treat respiratory infections.

- A quick and easy way of using garlic is to rub the inside of a salad bowl with a clove of raw garlic before adding the salad leaves.

55 feed your immune system

Hippocrates is credited with saying "let food be thy medicine and medicine be thy food". Support the immune system to stay strong and eat a healthy diet – it will increase the body's resistance to colds.

A healthy diet contains plenty of fresh fruit and vegetables, wholegrains, nuts and seeds. If you eat meat and/or fish, include a little chicken, turkey, game, lean red meat, shellfish and oily fish such as salmon, mackerel, herrings and tuna. Meat-eaters and vegetarians alike should include soya bean products, such as tofu or tempeh. Soya is a perfect source of protein.

Include plenty of raw food in your diet as all forms of cooking reduce some of the nutritional qualities.

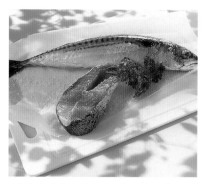

▲ Eat oily fish such as mackerel or salmon.

broccoli, mushroom and tofu salad
Marinate 250g/9oz firm tofu cubes for at least 1 hour in a mixture made up of 1 crushed garlic clove, 2.5cm/1in grated fresh root ginger, 45ml/3 tbsp each of soy sauce, tamari soy

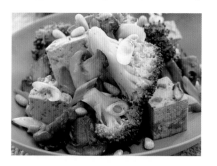

sauce and Chinese rice wine or dry sherry, 1.5m/¼ tsp each of cumin seeds and caster (superfine) sugar, and ground black pepper. Then stir-fry 1 finely chopped garlic clove over low heat for 1 minute, add 350g/12oz sliced mushrooms and cook over high heat for 4–5 minutes. Add 250g/9oz steamed broccoli florets and 4 thinly sliced spring onions (scallions) and season with pepper. Toss the tofu and marinade with the broccoli and mushrooms and serve sprinkled with pine nuts.

◄ Recent research suggests that soya offers protection against certain diseases.

56 easy breathing

Every year, more and more people are suffering from respiratory disorders, including colds, congested sinuses and chronic catarrh. These problems can be made worse by certain foods.

During a cold or respiratory infection, avoid sugar, cheese and dairy products, and processed, refined foods. This means saying "no" to white bread, pasta, cakes, pizza, any fast-food, and many commercial preparations, which tend to be highly processed and very often contain sugar. All of these foods encourage the production of mucus, which adds to the congestion in an overloaded respiratory system.

Tea, coffee, fizzy drinks and alcohol are also best avoided as they have a weakening effect on the immune system. Try fresh juices, herbal teas and plenty of mineral water instead.

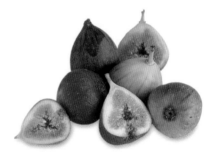

▲ Many fresh and dried fruits and berries, including figs, have antiviral properties.

easy breathing tips
To keep the lungs and airways healthy, eat plenty of unrefined, unprocessed foods. Additionally there are certain foods that seem to have a protective action on the respiratory system. Green vegetables, such as broccoli, peas, spinach and watercress are a good source of immunity boosting antioxidants. Carrots, sweet potatoes, apricots and mangoes are all high in betacarotene, from which the body can obtain vitamin A, which is anti-

infective and supports the mucus membranes. Eating plenty of citrus fruits, rich in vitamin C, together with onions, garlic, ginger and chilli will all help to open the airways and clear out mucus.

During a cold, avoid mucus-forming foods (these include dairy products and refined carbohydrates) and maintain a regular intake of garlic, ideally fresh. Garlic not only helps to stimulate the removal of excess mucus, but is one of the most powerful anti-infective agents available.

57 carrot revitalizer

Nutritious and easy to prepare, home-made juices are 100% pure, with nothing added or taken away. They are packed with essential vitamins and minerals and are excellent immunity boosters.

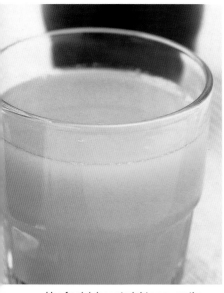

▲ *Use fresh juices straight away, as they lose their potency if they are left standing.*

Fresh carrots are one of nature's wonderfoods and are ideal for juicing. They are easy to obtain all the year round and are packed with vitamins. A single carrot is so rich in betacarotene that it provides an adequate daily intake of vitamin A, the vitamin that is necessary to maintain resistance against respiratory

infections. It is also high in vitamins C and E, with vitamin E also protecting the lungs against pollution and respiratory infections.

carrot, apple and orange juice
Carrot juice has a mild sweet taste, which mixes well with other fruit and vegetable juices. Try it with orange and apple juice, both fruits that are high in vitamin C. To make enough for one serving, take three carrots, scrubbed and trimmed, one apple, washed and cut into quarters, and an orange which has been peeled and cut into segments. Using a juice extractor, juice the carrots and fruit and pour into a glass. Serve immediately and drink by sipping slowly.

> Make fresh fruit and vegetable juices a regular part of your healthy eating plan. They support the immune system, are easy to digest, and help keep the body clean and free of toxins. They are packed with energy and healing properties – and they taste good too.

Squeeze citrus fruits and drink the juice neat or diluted with water to ward off a cold and ease a sore throat.

59

stimulating ginger

Ginger is widely used in traditional Chinese medicine to treat chills, fever, headaches and aching muscles, and the early European herbalists also recognized it as a cure for colds.

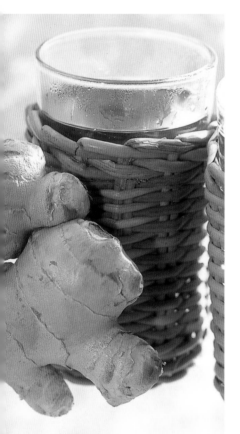

Ginger is a powerful immunity booster whose antiseptic, warming, anti-inflammatory and invigorating properties make it an invaluable medicine for the treatment of colds. This fiery spice stimulates the circulation and restores vitality, promoting feelings of wellbeing. It is especially useful during the long, cold, damp months of winter.

immunity-boosting lunch
Always make sure you have a supply of fresh ginger root available in the kitchen and get into the habit of using it in your cooking. A little fresh ginger root is delicious grated into a raw carrot salad. Try it for an immunity-boosting lunch – it will give you lots of energy for the afternoon.

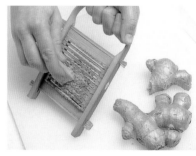

▲ ▸ *Ginger encourages the body to eliminate toxins, it opens up the nasal passages and has an expectorant action on the lungs.*

60 warming cayenne

The scarlet fruit pods (chillies) of the cayenne pepper plant have medicinal and culinary uses. The pods may be used whole or crushed to make powder, and are antibacterial and rich in vitamin C.

The heat of cayenne makes it useful as a strengthening tonic for the immune system and for warding off winter blues, lethargy and chills. Both the pods and the powder are powerful stimulants, boosting poor circulation and bringing warmth and vitality to the whole body. In particular, cayenne is excellent for treating the respiratory system. It is a powerful decongestant and expectorant and its pungency encourages the airways to open up, helping to alleviate the symptoms of a stuffy cold.

For general good health, try adding fresh chillies or cayenne powder to soups, curries and stews. To treat a cold or sore throat, add a pinch of cayenne powder to lemon juice, dilute with hot water and sweeten with honey. Drink three times daily.

CAUTIONS
- Extract the seeds from fresh chillies as these can be toxic.

- Avoid therapeutic doses of cayenne during pregnancy and while you are breastfeeding.

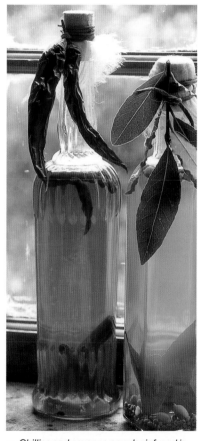

▲ Chillies and cayenne powder infused in cider vinegar make an effective medicine for treating the symptoms of a cold.

61 comforting cinnamon

For thousands of years, cinnamon has been used in the treatment of colds and flu. It warms and energizes the body, helping to ward off infection, and combat the listless feeling so typical of flu.

Cinnamon is a potent antiseptic, tonic and stimulant, which possesses antispasmodic properties. This sweetly pungent spice is taken from the inner bark of the cinnamon tree and is available as a brownish powder, or as small, delicately rolled sticks.

The bark of cinnamon promotes sweating and is ideal for treating "cold" conditions in the body, helping to relieve the aches and chills in the early stages of a cold or flu. Cinnamon sticks are often added to fruit punches in the winter for their warm, spicy aroma and their comforting effect.

The distinctive flavour and aroma of cinnamon combines well with oranges, which are rich in vitamin C. To make yourself a delicious hot toddy, add a stick of cinnamon to a glass of freshly squeezed orange juice. Top up with hot water and sweeten with honey. This health-giving drink should help to beat the winter blues and fight off infection.

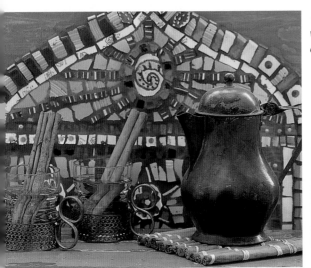

◄ *A hot orange tea flavoured with cinnamon makes a delicious drink to treat a cold.*

A centrally heated atmosphere can be a breeding ground for germs. Make sure you have enough fresh air and exercise to help the immune system stay strong.

62 soothing liquorice

Liquorice root has a cooling, soothing effect on mucus membranes. Its antispasmodic and expectorant action helps the airways to open up and expel or disperse any phlegm.

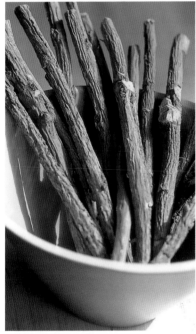

▲ Liquorice root is traditionally used to treat a wide range of respiratory problems.

In ancient Greece, liquorice was taken for asthma, chest problems and mouth ulcers – often a sign of being run down. Liquorice contains a substance 50 times sweeter than sugar, which stimulates the adrenals and encourages the body to produce its own hydrocortisone. In modern medicine, hydrocortisone is an important drug that is used to treat serious inflammatory conditions, including chronic chest problems.

liquorice cough tea

Dried liquorice root is generally available in good health stores. This can be boiled up in the proportion of 115g/4oz piece of dried liquorice root to 600ml/1 pint/2½ cups water to make a soothing tea. Alternatively, a few unsweetened black liquorice sticks can be covered in boiling water and left to dissolve. This will produce a strong extract that can be used to ease a chesty cough.

The dried, woody root of the liquorice plant is not only widely used in confectionery but has a tradition of medicinal use stretching back thousands of years. In Chinese medicine, liquorice is known as the "great detoxifier" as it is thought to drive poisons from the system.

63 elderflower tisane

Increasing fluid intake during a cold helps the body decongest and eliminate toxins. Tea, coffee and caffeinated drinks are best avoided and can be substituted with herb and spice teas instead.

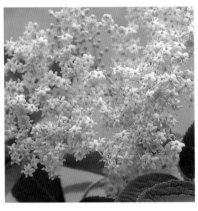

◄ *Elderflowers have been valued for their medicinal uses for thousands of years.*

Although you can buy herbal teas ready-made, making them fresh increases their health-giving properties. An easy way of making herbal teas is as an infusion or tisane, when the fresh or dried leaves, stems or flowers of a plant are left to steep in near-boiling water, which is then strained off and drunk.

A tisane of elderflower, chamomile and peppermint will help relieve many symptoms of a feverish cold. Peppermint has cooling properties and a stimulating, decongestant action. This is attributed to its high menthol content, making it particularly effective for clearing blocked sinuses and a stuffy nose. Elderflowers have anticatarrhal properties and encourage sweating, helping a fever to "come out", while chamomile flowers have a gentle anti-inflammatory, antispasmodic action and are a natural sedative. They are useful for bringing a fever down, soothing a racking and persistent cough, and promoting rest and sleep.

elderflower cold cure

To make the tea, the fresh or dried plant constituents may be used. You will need 2.5ml/½ tsp of each herb per 250ml/8fl oz/1 cup of near-boiling water. For fresh flowers and leaves, double up the quantities of each herb. Add the herbs to the hot water and leave to infuse for 5–10 minutes. Strain the liquid off and gently reheat if necessary. Pour into a mug and add a slice of lemon and a little honey to sweeten. For an extra warming effect, add a sprinkling of ground ginger. Drink the tea two or three times a day to combat a cold.

64 horehound infusion

Herbal teas are warm and comforting to drink and can help to ward off coughs and colds. They also bring relief from unpleasant symptoms – horehound can ease a feverish cold and a chesty cough.

The bitter juice extracted from the flowers and leaves of white horehound is an expectorant and a soothing tonic for the mucus membranes, making it a traditional cough medicine ingredient. Horehound is also a mild stimulant; it can relieve the groggy feeling that accompanies a bad cold.

horehound cough tea

Add some chopped fresh or dried leaves to 250ml/8fl oz/1 cup of near-boiling water. Infuse for 15 minutes, and strain off the liquid. Sweeten to taste with a little honey. This mixture may be drunk as a tea, three times daily between meals, or used as a gargle to alleviate a sore throat.

As well as being made into an infusion for drinking and gargling, horehound extract may be added to sugar syrup and boiled down to make cough candy.

▼ Drinking herbal teas is a good way to look after yourself when you have a cold.

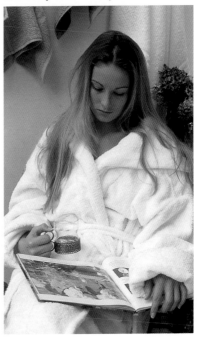

▼ Use horehound to ease a hacking cough.

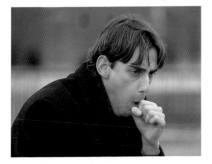

65

thyme infusion

In herbal medicine, thyme is recognized for its antiseptic properties and for its special affinity with the respiratory system. This makes it a valuable remedy for treating coughs and colds.

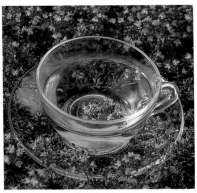

▲ An infusion made from thyme has a pungent taste, and its warming properties are good for treating chills.

Thyme contains the volatile oil, thymol, which has strong antiseptic, antifungal and antibacterial properties. These antiseptic properties make thyme a useful tonic for the immune system, as well as an effective remedy for chesty coughs and colds. Thyme has a powerful action on the respiratory system, producing expectoration and reducing bronchial spasm. It also has a warming, calming effect on the body and is useful during the chilly, shivering stage of a cold.

thyme cold treatment tea

Both the leaves and pink flowering tops can be used to make an infusion. For a brew, use 5ml/1 tsp dried thyme, or 10ml/2 tsp fresh, per 250ml/ 8fl oz/1 cup of near-boiling water. Steep the herbs in the water for 10 minutes, then drain off the liquid into a cup. Sweeten with honey if desired, add a slice of lemon and drink while hot. Drink the tea three times a day between meals.

▼ Relaxing quietly and keeping warm will help a cold clear up more quickly.

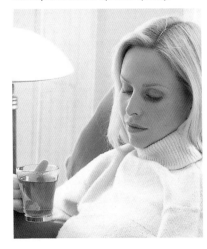

66 sage throat soother

A sore throat is often one of the first signs of a cold. Sage has powerful antiseptic, antibiotic and astringent properties and is useful for treating infections – particularly of the mouth and throat.

To ease a raspy throat, the juice of a freshly squeezed lemon combined with bitter sage leaves and sweetened with honey, produces a comforting, pleasant-tasting drink, packed with healing properties. Like sage, lemon is also a potent antiseptic and anti-inflammatory. This, together with its high vitamin C content, makes lemon a good choice for sore throats.

sage, honey & lemon tea

For a soothing tea, mix together 25g/ 1oz dried sage leaves with 30ml/ 2 tbsp clear honey. Add the freshly squeezed juice of a lemon, then dilute with 600ml/1 pint/2½ cups boiling water. Cover and leave to infuse for about 20–30 minutes. Strain into a non-aluminium pan and reheat the mixture until hot enough for drinking. Drink or gargle with the tea several times a day as needed.

CAUTIONS
- Avoid sage tea during pregnancy as it may stimulate uterine contractions.

- Thujone (an active ingredient of sage), can trigger fits in epileptics.

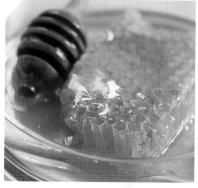

▲ Honey is also a natural antibiotic.

▼ Both lemon and sage are antiseptic.

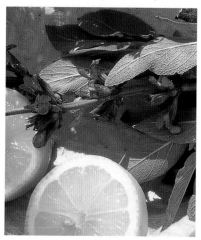

67

rosehip decoction

The high levels of vitamins and other nutrients found in rosehips are readily absorbed by the body. Rosehips should be picked when ripe and can be used fresh or dried to make delicious herbal teas.

Whole, dried rosehips will need softening and cooking in order to release their nutrients. This method of cooking herbs and spices to extract their therapeutic properties is known as decocting.

> Rosehips are good for you: a single rosehip typically contains 20 times more vitamin C than an average-sized orange.

▼ *Rosehip tea has a sweet astringent taste.*

rosehip cold cure

To make fresh rosehip tea, take 2–3 washed rosehips, top and tail them and leave them to soak overnight. Now fill a non-aluminium pan with 600ml/1 pint/2½ cups water and bring it to the boil. Add the rosehips and simmer for about 30 minutes. Finish by straining the mixture into a mug or cup, and add a little honey to sweeten if you wish. Drink the tea at intervals throughout the day – it will help the body to flush out toxins.

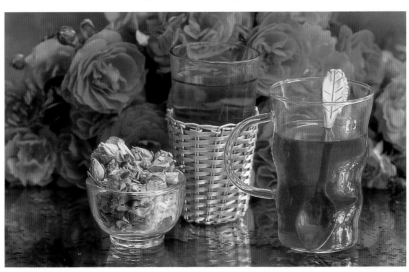

68 ginger & lemon tea

Keep ginger and lemon on standby for the onset of a shivery cold. Ginger is warming and stimulating and combines well with the sharp citrus tang of lemon to help the body fight off viral infections.

Decoctions are typically used to make medicinal concoctions from the root and bark of a plant. Ginger is extracted from the root of the ginger plant by boiling. The decoction lasts 2–3 days.

ginger and lemon decoction

To make a delicious hot ginger and lemon drink, take a 115g/4oz piece of washed fresh root ginger and slice it into 600ml/1 pint/2½ cups water in a non-aluminium pan. Take a lemon and grate it finely, adding the rind to the pan with a pinch of cayenne pepper. Bring the water to the boil, cover the pan and simmer for 20 minutes. Meanwhile, squeeze the rest of the lemon into a cup. When the ginger mixture has finished cooking, remove it from the heat and allow it to cool slightly before adding the lemon juice. Strain off the liquid, add honey to taste, and drink several times a day as needed.

Ginger stimulates the circulation, encouraging sweating, the elimination of toxins and the expulsion of mucus and catarrh.

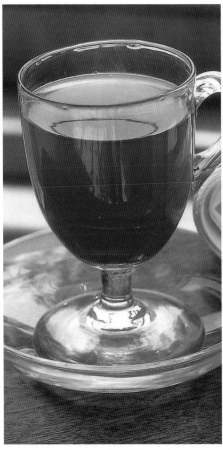

▲ *Enjoy a hot ginger and lemon toddy at bedtime – it's a traditional cold cure.*

hibiscus & rosehip tea

Hibiscus flowers have a soothing antispasmodic action, helpful for reducing fevers and soothing coughs. They combine well with rosehips – both plants are an excellent source of vitamin C.

Hibiscus flowers are a popular ingredient in many herbal teas. In Egypt, they form the basis of *karkade*, a chilled tea, traditionally served to travellers as a restorative after a long journey. Combined with rosehips, hibiscus makes a delicious, refreshing drink that is useful for treating cold symptoms or, better still, for keeping cold viruses at bay.

hibiscus and rosehip refresher
To make this soothing hibiscus and rosehip infusion, take two washed fresh rosehips. Top, tail and chop them up and place them in a bowl. Now add enough water to cover them, and leave to soak overnight. When the rosehip pieces are soft, strain off the water and add them to 5ml/1 tsp dried hibiscus flower petals. Add 250ml/8fl oz/ 1 cup of near-boiling water, cover and leave to infuse. When the mixture is ready, strain it into a non-aluminium pan and reheat until hot enough to drink. Pour the tea into a cup and sweeten with a little honey to taste. Drink regularly throughout the day as required.

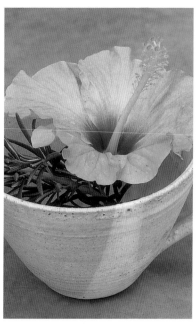

▲ *Hibiscus flowers are a delicious pick-me-up with many health-giving properties.*

CAUTION
Hibiscus *rosa-sinensis* is the medicinal variety, and should not be confused with the ornamental Hibiscus *sino-chinensis*, which is not suitable for making tea.

70

nasturtium tisane

Nasturtium is a traditional remedy of the Peruvian Indians for coughs, colds and flu. European herbalists used it to treat a wide range of ills, including scurvy and respiratory complaints.

Nasturtium was helpful against scurvy because of its high vitamin C content, and modern research shows that fresh nasturtium leaves contain a natural antibiotic that is effective in treating respiratory conditions. Nasturtium has powerful antimicrobial and decongestant properties and a warming and stimulating action on the body. This pungent and bitter plant is a good blood cleanser, stimulating the liver and helping the elimination of toxins. In order to treat respiratory congestion, some modern-day herbalists recommend eating 3 fresh nasturtium leaves a day. You can also add nasturtium flowers to a salad for a decorative and nutritious effect.

nasturtium cleanser

If you prefer, you can take nasturtium as a tea, using either the fresh or dried leaves. To make an infusion, pour a cup of near-boiling water on 10ml/ 2 tsp fresh, chopped leaves, or 5ml/ 1 tsp of the dried leaves and leave to stand for 10–15 minutes. Strain and drink three times a day to relieve colds, catarrh and chest infections.

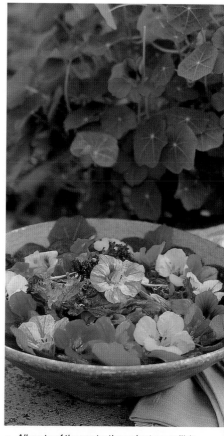

▲ *All parts of the nasturtium plant are edible and nutritious; nasturtium is rich in iron, vitamin C, minerals and trace elements.*

71

hyssop cold cleanser

Hyssop has been valued for thousands of years for its cleansing and purifying properties. It is a powerful antiseptic, excellent for warding off infection and strengthening the immune system.

The Cherokee Indians used the bitter leaves and delicate purple flowers of the hyssop plant to relieve respiratory disorders. Its expectorant and anticatarrhal properties, together

▾ *The fragrant flowers of the hyssop plant are much loved by bees and butterflies.*

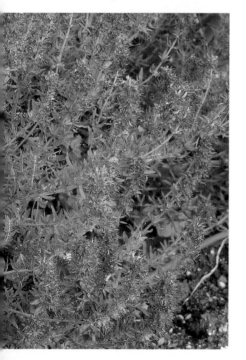

with a general affinity for the respiratory tract, make hyssop useful for treating coughs, colds and flu, plus associated disorders such as cold sores, catarrh, sinus problems and bronchitis. Additionally, hyssop has a warming and stimulating action on the circulatory system, helping to promote sweating, bring down fevers and cleanse the blood.

hyssop and orange tisane

The best way to take hyssop is in tea form. Add a few fresh or 5ml/1 tsp dried leaves and flowers to 250ml/ 8fl oz/1 cup of near-boiling water. Cover and leave to infuse for about 20–30 minutes. Strain into a non-aluminium pan and reheat the mixture until almost boiling. As hyssop is bitter, sweeten the tea with a little honey. For extra flavour, add a little freshly squeezed orange juice.

Hyssop has antiviral properties, and is useful for treating the herpes simplex virus, which causes cold sores. Dab a few drops of the tea on to a cotton pad at the first sign of itching.

lime blossom cooler

Lime blossom has a gentle, calming effect on the nervous system and is ideal for treating irritating, spasmodic coughs, soothing sore throats and bringing down a fever. Enjoy it as an infusion.

The yellow flowers of the lime or linden tree are acknowledged in folklore for their healing and restorative powers. When taken in a hot infusion, they help the body to sweat while cooling it down at the same time. This makes lime flower tea a good choice for feverish colds and flu.

lime blossom and peppermint tea
Put 5 or 6 fresh lime flowers (picked just as they open) or 1–3 tsp dried flower heads with a few fresh or dried peppermint leaves into a pot. Pour over to 250ml/8fl oz/1 cup of almost-boiling water. Cover and leave to infuse for 5–10 minutes. For a weaker brew, use 1 tsp of dried lime flowers and infuse for 4–5 minutes. Sweeten with honey to taste.

The gentle, soothing action of lime blossom makes it particularly suitable for treating children's coughs, colds and fevers. Use the weaker version of the tea omitting the peppermint and infusing for 4 minutes. Serve three times a day.

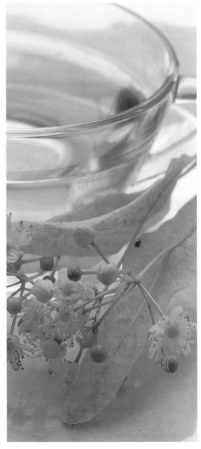

▲ *Lime blossom tisane has a delicate, pale lemon colour and a subtle taste.*

73 summer fruit cordial

Fruit cordials are a pleasant way to enjoy the health-giving properties of plants. Home-made ones will keep refrigerated for several months, stored in a screw-top bottle.

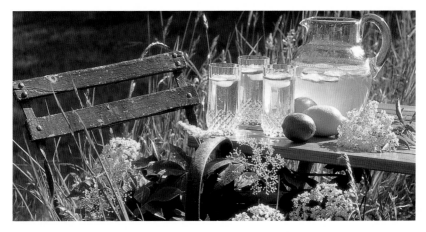

▲ *To avoid a summer cold, drink vitamin C-rich elderflower cordial.*

To treat a summer cold, try this deliciously refreshing elderflower and lime cordial: limes have a high vitamin C content and elderflowers are anticatarrhal. The drink is soothing on the throat and its zingy flavour will lift your spirits whenever you feel unwell. It will keep refrigerated for 2–3 months.

10 fresh elderflower heads
2–3 limes, sliced
675g/1½lb/3 cups sugar
5ml/1 tsp citric acid
5ml/1 tsp cream of tartar
1 litre/1¾ pints/4 cups boiling water

Wash and pick over the elderflowers thoroughly, discarding any that are past their best. Put them into a large bowl with the sliced limes. Add the sugar, citric acid and cream of tartar. Set aside for up to 12 hours. Pour in the boiling water and leave to stand for 24 hours. Strain the syrup into sterilized bottles and seal the contents with corks. To serve, dilute with about twice as much still or sparkling mineral water.

74 elderberry rob

Ripe elderberries are rich in vitamins A and C. They can be made into syrups and wines for preventing and treating coughs and colds, to bring down fevers and to soothe sore throats.

Elderberry is one of the oldest known medicinal herbs with expectorant and antiviral properties. Home-made elderberry cordial is easy to make and a useful standby for the winter season. The cordial can be diluted with hot or cold water and lemon juice to relieve a feverish cold and support the immune system, or taken neat as a cough and throat soother. During a cold, drink two or three glasses a day.

elderberry winter warmer
1kg/2¼lb elderberries
350g/12oz/1½ cups sugar
grated rind and juice of an orange
10 crushed coriander seeds
1 cinnamon stick

Put all the ingredients into a non-aluminium pan and heat gently until the sugar is dissolved. Let the mixture simmer over a low heat for 20 minutes. When the liquid has cooled, strain and pour into a sterilized screw-top bottle. The cordial will keep refrigerated for several months.

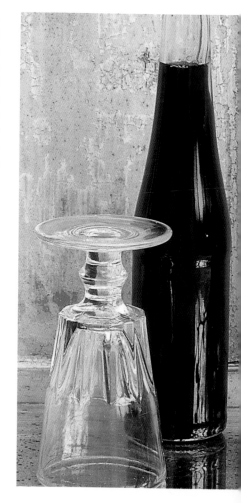

▸ *Elderberries are packed with health-giving properties to ease the symptoms of a cold.*

herbal cough linctus

The decongestant and expectorant action of borage makes it a traditional ingredient in cough syrup recipes. It combines well with the antiseptic properties of thyme.

Making your own cough syrup is quite an easy process. The following thyme and borage linctus will keep refrigerated for up to 2 months in a screw-top bottle. Take 5ml/1 tsp as needed to ease a dry, scratchy cough.

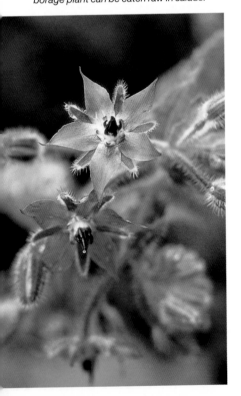

▼ The delicate star-shaped flowers of the borage plant can be eaten raw in salads.

thyme & borage linctus

25g/1oz fresh or 15g/½oz dried thyme
25g/1oz fresh or 15g/½oz dried
    borage flowers and leaves
2 x 5cm/2in cinnamon sticks
600ml/1 pint/2½ cups water
juice of 1 small lemon
100g/4oz/½ cup honey

Put the herbs into a non-aluminium pan with the cinnamon and water. Bring to the boil, cover and simmer for 20 minutes. Strain off the liquid and return to the pan. Simmer, uncovered, until the liquid is reduced by half. Stir in the lemon juice and honey and simmer gently for 5 minutes. Pour into a screw-top bottle and refrigerate.

The cooling and cleansing properties of borage make it useful for detoxifying the system and for any condition associated with excess heat.

sore throat gargle

Regular use of mouthwashes and gargles helps keep the mouth and throat germ-free. At the onset of a cold, gargle with an infusion of sage and thyme to ease the discomfort of a sore throat.

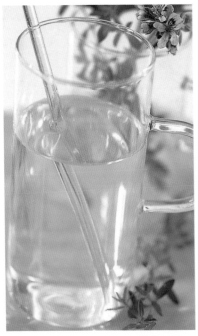

▲ Thyme fortifies the immune system in its fight against bacterial and viral infections.

Both thyme and sage are powerful antiseptics, sage having a particular affinity with the mouth and throat, and thyme with the chest and lungs. The two herbs together make a powerful combination for treating the symptoms of a cold, particularly sore throats and tickly coughs. If you are able to catch the symptoms quickly enough you may be able to prevent them from developing.

Making your own gargle or cough medicine is quick and easy using an infusion of fresh or dried herbs. Gargle with the mix three or four times a day, or take 10ml/2 tsp, three or four times a day as a soothing linctus.

thyme & sage gargle
small handful of fresh sage flowers and leaves or 30ml/2 tbsp dried herb
small handful of thyme flowers and leaves or 30ml/2 tbsp dried herb
600ml/1 pint/2½ cups boiling water
30ml/2 tbsp cider vinegar
10ml/2 tsp honey
5ml/1 tsp cayenne pepper

Place the fresh or dried herbs into a jug, pour in the boiling water, cover and leave to infuse for 30 minutes. Strain off the water and stir in the cider vinegar, honey and cayenne. Pour the mixture into a screw-top bottle and keep in a cool place. The mixture will keep for 1 week.

77

garlic & honey syrup

The compounds contained in garlic can help prevent and cure infection. Garlic is one of the most powerful natural remedies for treating coughs, colds and flu. Use it with honey to make a soothing cold cure.

Garlic has powerful antiseptic and antiviral properties and combines well with honey, which is soothing, to make a syrup to prevent or relieve cold and flu symptoms. Take 15ml/1 tbsp three times a day as a preventative, or to ease the first signs of a cold. The syrup will keep for up to 2–3 weeks in the refrigerator.

garlic cold cure
1 head of garlic
300ml/½ pint/1¼ cups water
juice of ½ lemon
30ml/2 tbsp honey

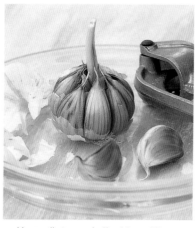

▲ Use garlic to ward off colds and flu.

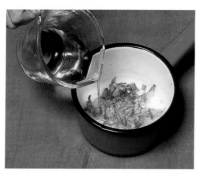

1 Wash and crush the garlic cloves – there is no need to peel them. Put them in a pan with the water. Bring to the boil, cover and simmer gently for 20 minutes.

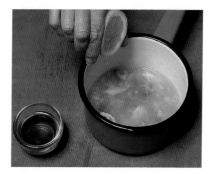

2 Add the lemon juice and honey and simmer for 2–3 minutes. Let the mixture cool, then strain it into a clean, dark glass jar or bottle with an airtight lid.

78 marshmallow soother

If left untreated, a heavy cold can turn into more serious health problems such as laryngitis or bronchitis. Use marshmallow to treat an acute sore throat, hoarseness and a dry, hacking cough.

The name of the marshmallow plant is derived from a Greek word meaning "to heal" and the plant is well known for its ability to soothe and heal bronchial disorders. The heart-shaped leaves and the soft pink flowers have a protective and soothing action on the mucus membranes: they both encourage the expulsion of phlegm and can relieve dry coughs, bronchial asthma, bronchial catarrh and pleurisy.

The following gargle combines marshmallow with cider vinegar, also known for its antiseptic and healing properties, and should help relieve a painful throat and dry, hacking cough. Use it three or four times a day, or take it as a linctus: 10ml/2 tsp, two or three times a day.

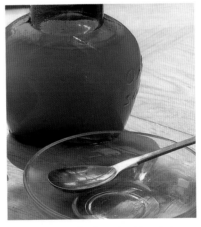

▲ Herbal remedies keep best in a dark glass bottle or jar with a tight-fitting lid.

marshmallow gargle
1 small handful of fresh marshmallow
   or 30ml/2 tbsp of the dried herb
600ml/1 pint/2½ cups boiling water
30ml/2 tbsp cider vinegar
30ml/2 tbsp honey

Add the fresh or dried marshmallow to a jug containing the boiling water. Cover and leave to infuse for up to 30 minutes and then strain off the herbs. Stir in the cider vinegar and the honey to taste. Pour the mixture into a dark bottle or jar with a screw-top lid. It will keep for up to 1 week stored in a cool place.

Infections of the upper respiratory tract should be taken seriously and treated as soon as possible. If they do not respond to home treatment, seek medical advice.

79

lavender balm

A sore, red nose, dry lips and cold sores often accompany a cold. These symptoms are best treated locally by the application of a soothing skin salve containing healing plant oils.

Beeswax and cocoa butter form a good basis for a salve. They are rich emollients and will help to moisturize the skin. Wheatgerm oil is high in vitamin E, and seems to work wonders when applied to dry skin. It also helps to preserve the cream.

Lavender is a good addition to a skin salve as it has antiseptic, antiviral and anti-inflammatory properties. Its antiviral properties are particularly useful for treating cold sores. The best way of using it in a cream is to add a few drops of the essential oil.

▾ *Lavender promotes the rapid healing of broken skin and soothes inflammation.*

lavender skin soother
5ml/1 tsp beeswax
5ml/1 tsp cocoa butter
5ml/1 tsp wheatgerm oil
5ml/1 tsp almond oil

Add the ingredients to a small bowl. Set the bowl over a pan of simmering water and stir the contents until the wax has melted.

Remove the bowl from the heat and allow the mixture to cool for a few minutes before adding 3 drops of lavender essential oil. Pour the mix into a small, screw-topped jar and leave to set. Store the cream away from the light and use as required.

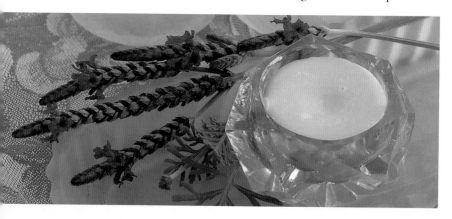

80 chest rub

A blocked nose is one of the most miserable aspects of having a cold. An old-fashioned back and chest rub with lavender and eucalyptus can work wonders to ease sinus congestion.

Lavender and eucalyptus used together make an effective decongestant rub. Eucalyptus is a traditional Aboriginal fever remedy, and the essential oil is one of the most antiseptic of herbal essences. The oil's aroma is both penetrating and refreshing, and an immune-system stimulant. Lavender also has powerful antiseptic and antibiotic properties, and a decongesting and expectorant action. It is also an effective sedative.

lavender and eucalyptus rub
50g/2oz petroleum jelly
15ml/1 tbsp dried lavender heads
6 drops eucalyptus essential oil
4 drops camphor essential oil

Melt the petroleum jelly in a bowl over a pan of simmering water. Stir in the lavender and heat for 30 minutes. Strain the liquid jelly through a piece of muslin and allow to cool before adding the essential oils. Pour the mix into a clean jar and leave until set.

Massage the rub on to the throat, chest and upper back at bedtime so the oils penetrate the skin and the vapours are inhaled throughout the night.

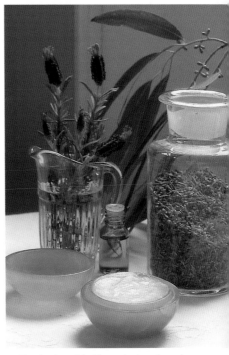

▲ Use fresh or dried lavender heads and eucalyptus oil in a chest and back rub.

> **CAUTION**
> Eucalyptus and camphor should be avoided if taking homeopathic treatment.

81   herbal compresses

Natural medicine sees fever as an important healing process. Herbal extracts can be applied to the body on hot or cold compresses to help bring the fever out and/or down.

Compresses are made by making a herbal infusion and then soaking a clean cloth in the hot water. The cloth is then wrung out and either applied to the body while it is still warm or left to cool before applying.

hot compress

Chamomile, cypress, juniper, lavender, peppermint, tea tree and rosemary will all induce sweating if the body needs to sweat. Drop a handful of fresh or dried herbs into a basin of hot water and leave to infuse for 5–10 minutes. Soak a clean cloth in the water, wring it out and use while hand-hot as needed.

cold compress

Bergamot, eucalyptus, lavender and peppermint have a cooling effect on the body and are useful to bring a fever down when it is dangerously high. Again, make an infusion with a handful of fresh or dried herbs dropped into a basin of hot water and leave to infuse as before. Let the water cool before soaking a clean cloth in it. Wring out the cloth and apply to the forehead or the back of the neck.

Lavender and peppermint have a balancing action on the body and can be used for both hot and cold compresses.

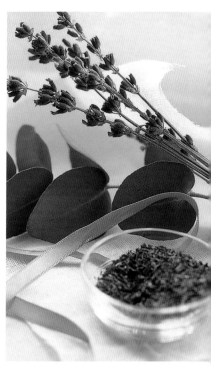

▲ Eucalyptus and lavender are effective on a cool compress to bring a fever down.

82

elderflower tincture

Tinctures have a reasonably long shelf-life and are an effective way to extract the active ingredients of plants. They can be made with fresh or dried plant material steeped in a mixture of alcohol and water.

The creamy white blossoms of the elder tree are an excellent remedy for the onset of colds and flu. At the first signs of discomfort − aching, sore throat, chills, restlessness and fever − elderflowers will stimulate the system and cause sweating. Sweating cleanses the body, eliminating toxins via the pores of the skin, and is the body's way of throwing off infection. Elderflowers also have a relaxing and decongestant action on the bronchi, reducing muscle spasm and also helping to expel any phlegm.

You can benefit from the healing properties of elderflowers all the year round by making them into a tincture. Preserved in an alcohol base, the tincture will keep for up to 2 years. Since tinctures are highly concentrated extracts, you should not exceed a dosage of more than 5ml/1 tsp, three or four times a day. You can dilute your elderflower tincture in a little water or add to your favourite fruit juice if preferred.

▸ *The anticatarrhal properties of elder tree blossoms make them an excellent choice for making a cold-cure tincture.*

cold-cure tincture
15g/½ oz dried elderflowers
250ml/8fl oz/1 cup vodka
    made up to 300ml/½ pint/1¼ cups
    with water

Put the dried elderflowers into a glass jar and pour in the vodka and water mixture. Seal the jar and leave in a cool, dark place for 7–10 days (no longer), shaking occasionally. Strain off the elderflowers through a sieve lined with kitchen paper before pouring the mixture into a sterilized bottle. Store in a cool, dark place.

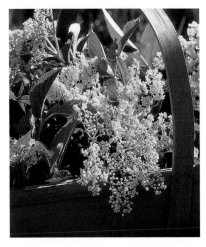

83 rose petal tonic

Rose leaves and petals have a cooling effect, which is useful for bringing down a fever and clearing heat and toxins from the body. Preserve their healing properties in a medicinal vinegar.

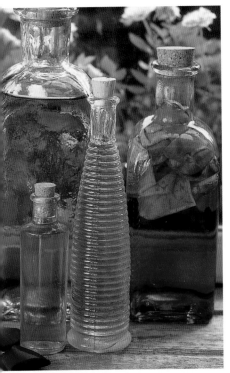

▲ *Rose petal vinegar is a tonic for a cold.*

Raspberry vinegar, made with 115g/4oz raspberries and 600ml/ 1 pint/2½ cups cider vinegar is useful for treating sore throats.

Cider vinegar is the preferred choice for making a medicinal vinegar. It is an antiseptic and has a balancing action on the body. Dried or fresh rose leaves and petals are then added to the vinegar and left to steep.

The soothing, astringent action of rose petals is strengthening to the lungs and is useful for relieving cold and flu symptoms, easing a sore throat and drying up a runny nose. Rose also has an uplifting effect on the spirits and can ease a headache.

rose petal vinegar
50g/2oz fresh rose petals
600ml/1 pint/2½ cups cider vinegar

For a soothing rose vinegar, put the ingredients in a screw-top jar. Screw on the lid and leave in a warm place for 10 days. Strain off the liquid into a sterilized seal-top container and store in a cool, dark place.

The vinegar may be used as a gargle for the throat or taken as a linctus: 5ml/1 tsp, three or four times a day. Alternatively, dab a few drops on to a tissue and apply to the temples to ease a feverish headache.

four thieves remedy

This traditional recipe is attributed to a gang of four thieves who avoided catching the plague in medieval France by making liberal use of a strong herbal vinegar. Try it to guard against colds and flu.

Many versions of the recipe have been attributed to the four thieves. This formula, based on an amalgam of the old recipes, is effective as a mild antiseptic, or to take in prophylactic doses of 5ml/1 tsp, two or three times a day, when exposed to colds and other viral infections. The recipe benefits from the health-giving properties of cider vinegar.

four thieves vinegar
15ml/1 tbsp each dried lavender,
  rosemary, sage and peppermint
2–3 bay leaves
10ml/2 tsp dried wormwood
5ml/1 tsp garlic granules
5ml/1 tsp ground cloves
5ml/1 tsp ground cinnamon
600ml/1 pint/2½ cups cider vinegar

Put all the dry ingredients into a jar and fill it with the cider vinegar. Cover tightly and leave in a warm place, such as on a sunny windowsill or by a central heating boiler, for 10 days. Strain off the liquid, through a sieve lined with kitchen paper, into a clean jug. Finally, pour the vinegar into a sterilized bottle and seal.

▼ *Ingredients for Four Thieves Vinegar (clockwise from right): lavender and bay, rosemary, peppermint, cloves, cinnamon and wormwood, garlic and sage.*

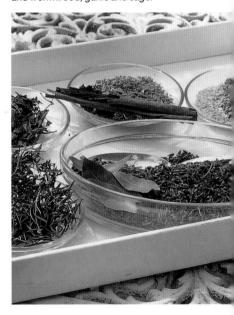

CAUTIONS
• Do not take internally for more than 2 weeks at a time.

• Do not take if pregnant, as wormwood is a uterine stimulant.

85 allium inhalant

For centuries, steam inhalations have been used to ease problems in the respiratory tract, including coughs, colds, sinus congestion and sore throats. Garlic has beneficial antiseptic properties.

Very hot steam is in itself a hostile environment for viruses and works well with the antibacterial and antiviral action of the oils to kill off many germs. To make the most out of

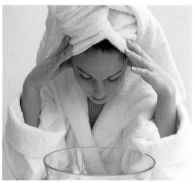

▲ Pour boiling water into a bowl containing garlic or another herb and inhale the steam.

a steam inhalation, have the steam as hot as you can bear without actually burning your nose and throat as you breathe in.

steam inhalant with garlic

The antiseptic properties of garlic will help to ease a sore throat. Put two unpeeled garlic cloves in a heatproof bowl containing 1 litre/1¼ pints/4 cups of steaming hot water. Lean over the bowl, covering your head a with a towel to make a tent over the bowl. Sit in the steam and inhale the garlic aroma for 5-10 minutes, or for as long as is comfortable.

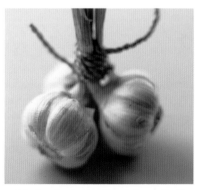

▲ Inhaling the aroma of garlic is an effective way to clear the nasal passages.

CAUTION
Inhalations should be carefully monitored if you are asthmatic or suffer from hay fever or any allergy. If this is the case, they should only be used for up to 1 minute; providing this provokes no adverse reaction, the time can gradually be increased up to 3–5 minutes.

86

essential oils

Essential oils capture the essence of the plant and all its healing properties in a highly concentrated form. Aromatherapy describes the use of these oils for therapeutic purposes.

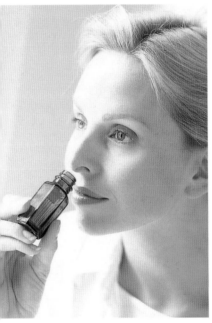

▲ Inhaling an essential oil is a quick way of enjoying its health-giving properties.

Aromatherapy works by inhalation and/or by absorption into the skin. With one or two exceptions, oils are never put directly on to the skin but are added to a suitable carrier base, such as water (for bathing) or vegetable oil (for massage).

aromatherapy cold cures

There are many essential oils that can be comforting and helpful for a cold. Some of the most effective include tea tree and eucalyptus, which have a long tradition of use in Aboriginal medicine. Both oils are powerful antiseptics with a clean and penetrating "medicinal" aroma.

Peppermint, rosemary, lavender, frankincense, sandalwood and jasmine are also useful for a cold. Peppermint and rosemary have a fresh, uplifting aroma, which can help to clear blocked sinuses and relieve a stuffy head cold. Lavender is an antiviral and an immunity booster; it also soothes inflammation and restores balance to the body.

Frankincense and sandalwood are especially good for easing congestion in chesty coughs and colds, and jasmine oil is also useful for treating catarrh and chest infections.

CAUTION
Essential oils are not for internal use and should be handled with care and respect.

87 warming foot baths

A foot bath can restore and revitalize the whole body. Add mustard or essentials oils for a relaxing and therapeutic experience that will help combat the symptoms of a head cold or feverish chill.

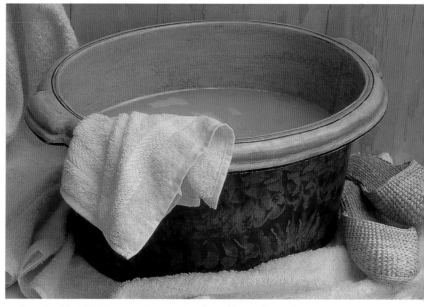

▲ *A mustard foot bath is a popular treatment for colds and flu that has stood the test of time.*

A hot foot bath has an immediate invigorating effect on the body. The warmth of the water helps the blood vessels to dilate, which in turn relaxes the body and improves circulation, helping to combat fluey chills. The addition of mustard or a suitable essential oil to the water will enhance the overall effect.

mustard foot bath

Black mustard is a well-known spice, but its main therapeutic use is as an external application. Mustard has a warming, stimulating effect on the circulation, encouraging sweating and relieving muscular aches and pains. Indulged in at the onset of a cold or chill, this easy-to-prepare foot bath using mustard powder will have a warming and comforting effect on the whole body.

Pour 2.2 litres/4 pints/9 cups hot water into a large heatproof bowl. Add 15ml/1 tbsp mustard powder to the water and stir in well until it is dissolved. Immerse the feet while the bath is still hot, but not burning, and sit back and relax for 20–30 minutes. Keep topping up the bowl with hot water if necessary.

using essential oils

A foot bath containing a few drops of essential oil is a quick and effective way to soothe muscular aches or stimulate the circulation to warm up a shivery body or chilled feet. Simply add 3–4 drops of your chosen oils to a large bowl two-thirds full of hot water. Because the heat of the water will release the therapeutic effect of the oils immediately, you should have everything ready for the treatment before you add the oil.

Several essential oils are useful for easing many unpleasant cold and flu symptoms. As well as the beneficial properties absorbed through the skin, the released aromas will help to relax and soothe as they are breathed in. A blend of 2 drops each of rosemary and marjoram or pine oils will work wonders for muscular aches and pains. To improve circulation and warm up cold extremities use 2 drops each of lavender and marjoram oils.

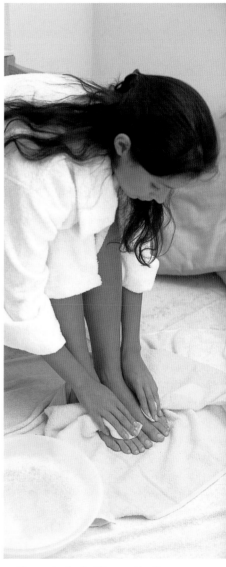

▲ Always dry the feet thoroughly after treatment, especially between the toes, to prevent problems such as athlete's foot.

aromatic inhalations

A steam inhalation warms and moistens the airways. Adding essential oils helps to open and relax the airways, clearing the congested nasal passages and soothing the mucus membranes.

For an inhalation to relieve a stuffy head cold, a combination of eucalyptus and tea tree oil is ideal. Studies show that tea tree oil is active against all types of infectious organisms: bacteria, fungi and viruses. It is also a very powerful immune stimulant, increasing the body's ability to respond to these organisms. Eucalyptus also has a powerful antibacterial and antiviral action, and its sharply penetrating aroma is well known as a decongestant.

eucalyptus and tea tree inhalation
Boil a kettle and pour approximately 600ml/1 pint/2½ cups hot water into a large heatproof bowl – one the size of a washing-up bowl is ideal. Add 3 drops of tea tree and 2 drops of eucalyptus to the water. Sit in front of the bowl with a towel draped over your head and shoulders to form a tent. As the oils vaporize, breathe in the steam as deeply as possible; take the steam as hot as you can bear it without burning your nose or throat. The action of the oils should begin to decongest blocked nasal passages, kill off the germs and soothe the unpleasant cold symptoms.

If you prefer, rosemary and peppermint oils may be substituted to achieve a similar result.

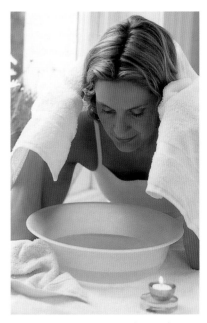

▲ Inhaling steam scented with eucalyptus or tea tree oil is a powerful antiseptic that will help to decongest blocked sinuses.

massage for colds

The power of touch to comfort and bring healing to the body is widely recognized. Essential oils can be used in an upper back and chest massage to make a relaxing and effective cold treatment.

Massage is not only relaxing and a good tension-easer, it also boosts the immune system and helps the body to eliminate toxins. When using essential oils in massage, they must be added to a suitable massage oil or unperfumed cream/lotion base. High-quality vegetable oils, such as sunflower, almond or wheatgerm, are ideal as

▾ *Massage stimulates the circulation and encourages the elimination of toxins.*

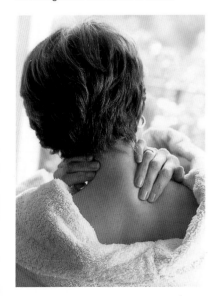

a massage base oil. Use a total of 4–5 drops of essential oil to 30ml/ 2 tbsp base oil, lotion or cream.

selecting an essential oil
There are many essential oils that can help a cold, particularly tea tree, peppermint, lavender and eucalyptus. Additionally, marjoram can ease a tickly cough and chest congestion, and myrrh is also helpful for thick catarrh and a whooping-type cough. If the cold has given way to laryngitis, try a combination of sandalwood, niaouli and lemon grass oils massaged on to the upper back and chest.

upper back and chest massage
To give the massage, gently spread the oil across the upper back and chest and work it into the skin. On the back, this can be done with a wide stroking movement, on the front use small circular movements with the tips of the fingers. Notice any areas that feel particularly tight or tender and give them an extra working. If you don't have anyone to give you a back massage, the treatment is equally effective as an upper chest rub.

90 quick decongestant

Almost any part of the body benefits from being massaged. To ease sinus congestion, a gentle facial self-massage will encourage drainage of mucus from the nose and sinuses.

The massage can be done with or without essential oils. Select the oils according to your symptoms. If there is a dull pain in the forehead and sinus cavities, lavender and thyme are effective, whereas tea tree, eucalyptus, peppermint and pine are all good at clearing congestion. Add 4–5 drops of the combined essential oils to 30ml/2 tbsp of massage oil. The following routine is best done after an aromatic steam inhalation, which will have opened up the airways and softened the mucus.

sinus self-massage

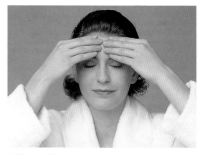

1 Start all over your brow, beginning at the centre and working out with small circular motions from your fingertips.

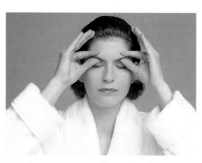

2 Release pressure from the sinus passages by pinching along the ridge of your eyebrows with your thumbs and index fingers, starting on the inside corners and working, step by step, to the outer edge.

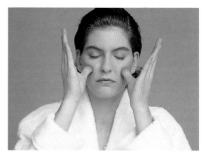

3 The small indentations beneath the ridges of the cheekbones indicate the site of some of the sinus passages. Apply thumb pressure slowly up into the hollows. Hold for a count of five and release. This will help to clear the head.

91 bathing with oils

Bathing with essential oils is one of the simplest and yet most effective aromatherapy treatments. An aromatic bath can help to detoxify the body and ease the symptoms of colds and viral infections.

Essential oils have a dual action in the bath: they are absorbed through the skin into the bloodstream, while their aromas are inhaled, working directly on the senses and emotions.

baths for a cold

There are many different oils that are suitable for treating coughs, colds and flu. Fill the bath first with comfortably hot water then add the essential oil(s) just before you get in, swirling the water round to disperse them. To avoid an oily scum around the bath, you can mix them together first in a little milk or add them to an unscented foam bubble bath.

Pamper yourself with an aromatic bath.

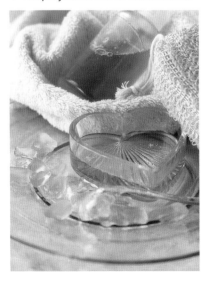

- At the first sign of a cold, bathing with tea tree oil can often stop the cold developing. Run a hot bath and swish 2–3 drops of the oil to the water.

- For a cold with a cough, a combination of rosemary, sage and peppermint will make an energizing morning bath. Add 1 drop of each oil to the water.

- A fluey cold will benefit from a rosemary, peppermint and ginger mix. Add 1 drop of each oil to a morning bath.

- When convalescing after a heavy cold, enjoy a relaxing evening bath with 2 drops of lavender, 1 drop rose and 1 drop ylang ylang oil.

winter warmer

In the shivery, aching, hot-and-cold stage of a feverish cold or flu, a hand bath may be a preferable option to a full-body bath. Add essential oils of ginger and nutmeg to warm the body.

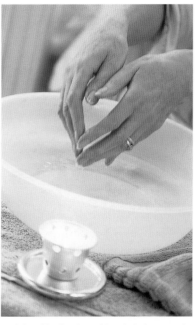

▲ A hand bath using a blend of ginger and nutmeg oil will help ease a fluey cold.

The essential oils of nutmeg and ginger are useful for treating a shivery, runny-nosed winter cold. Similar to cinnamon, nutmeg oil has a stimulating effect on the body, helping to warm and tone it up and build resistance to colds. Ginger is also a stimulating, warming oil and useful for colds. Similar to the fresh root, its fiery properties are useful for treating any condition associated with excess damp; it heats up the body and helps to dry out excess moisture.

warming hand bath

To make a hand bath, fill a large bowl two-thirds full with hot water. Add 1 drop of each essential oil and swish the water before sitting back with your hands in the bowl. Soak your hands for 10–15 minutes. The warmth of the water will help the blood vessels in your hands to dilate and the body to relax, while the oils are absorbed into the bloodstream.

CAUTIONS
- Ginger and nutmeg oils should be used with care as they may cause a skin reaction in some individuals. If in doubt, do a skin-patch test first on the inside of the wrist or elbow.

- Do not use nutmeg oil if you are pregnant or breastfeeding.

Add a few drops of

lavender oil to a

cool compress to

ease aching limbs and

a hot, burning headache.

homeopathic cures

Homeopathy views symptoms as the body's attempt to heal itself. A homeopathic remedy is selected on the basis of a "picture" of these symptoms, which will vary between individuals.

Most homeopathic remedies are prepared from a tincture of an original plant or mineral substance. This is then diluted many times, until barely a trace of the original substance remains. Instead, the remedy is thought to contain an "energy blueprint" of the original substance, which then works on the body's energy system, to stimulate the self-healing process.

selecting a cold remedy

As homeopathic treatment is unique to the individual, choose the remedy that best fits with your "symptom-picture". Take three times a day in the 6C potency or once a day in the 30C potency until symptoms improve.

▼ *Homeopathic remedies are available as a small, tasteless pill, or as drops.*

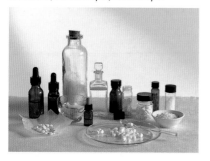

ACONITE: symptoms that come on suddenly, often at night. Flu is marked by profuse sweating and a high fever.

ALLIUM CEPA or *ARSENICUM*: at the first sign of a head cold, try either of these two remedies. Allium cepa is marked by watery eyes and a runny nose, and Arsenicum by looking pale and feeling chilly.

BELLADONNA: symptoms that come on quickly with a high fever, marked by redness, burning heat and a throbbing headache.

BRYONIA: symptoms come on more slowly, accompanied by extreme thirst, irritability and the desire to be left alone.

GELSEMIUM: this is the most widely used flu remedy. The most pronounced symptoms are shaking with shivering, aching muscles and general weakness.

FERRUM PHOS: for symptoms that are not well defined or as a general tonic during and after the flu.

reiki healing

Reiki is a Japanese healing system based on channelling healing energy to the body. Receiving reiki is a relaxing experience and can help with common ailments such as coughs and colds.

Reiki healing can bring rapid relief from a common cold; the subtle healing energy is so effective, that symptoms have been known to clear up almost instantaneously. Reiki works by putting the hands in certain positions on the body and then allowing the healing energy to flow through them.

Reiki is learned by being initiated or "attuned" by a Reiki Master. Reiki classes are widely available.

reiki cold treatment

To give a reiki treatment, stand to one side of the recipient and place one hand on the forehead and your other hand on the centre of the chest. This will help relieve a headache, an aching neck and shoulders, blocked airways and coughing. The position of the hand on the chest is also comforting and relaxing.

Leave the hands in this position until you feel it's enough. Then move to stand behind the recipient and place the fingers of both hands under the cheekbones. This will help to ease congestion in the sinuses.

▸ *A reiki treatment can have many therapeutic and healing benefits for both the practitioner and the receiver.*

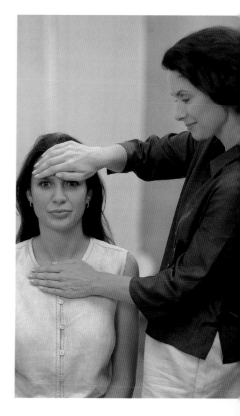

reflexology treatments

By applying gentle pressure to certain points on the feet, reflexology stimulates the body to heal itself. Reflexology can boost the immune system and treat colds, sore throats and sinus problems.

The ball of each foot represents one side of your chest. Here lie the reflexes to vital respiratory organs such as the lungs, air passages, heart, thymus gland, as well as to the breast and shoulders. The whole area is bounded by the diaphragm, the reflex that lies across the ball of each foot.

To treat a cold with blocked or painful sinuses, you need to give all the toes a good working as this is where the sinus reflexes are situated. After treatment, drink plenty of water to flush out the toxins that have been displaced, and keep yourself warm.

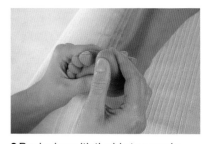

2 Beginning with the big toe, apply firm pressure to the tops of all the toes. This will help to clear the sinuses. Then pinpoint the pituitary gland in the centre of the prints of both big toes to stimulate the endocrine system.

cold treatment routine

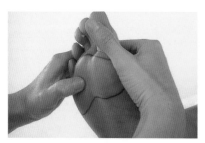

1 Begin by working the whole chest area. This will help the airways open up and encourage clear breathing.

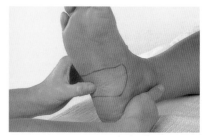

3 Treat the upper lymph system by working down the front of the toes to stimulate the immune system. Then work the large area above the heel to stimulate the small intestines and colon. This helps the body to eliminate toxins.

sore throat treatment

This nasty by-product of a cold or cough can be treated by giving the whole chest area a thorough workout. The thymus and lymph glands are among the body's chief mechanisms for fighting off infection, and regular attention to these areas via reflexology treatment will help to ward off future illnesses. This sore throat soother also encourages stimulation of the immune system and adrenal glands, to prompt these similarly vital infection-fighters to respond to the virus.

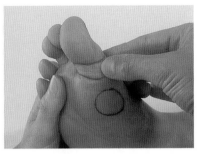

1 Work the upper lymph system (shown here at the edge of the joint of the big toe), then work the throat via the neck reflex at the centre of the pad. Work the thymus gland (circled) to encourage the immune system to respond.

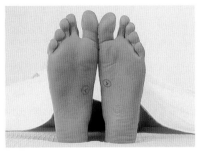

3 Work the adrenal reflex by applying pressure to the ball of each foot, in the direction of the arrow. This will help to reduce inflammation.

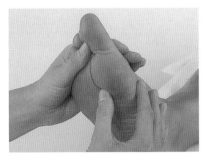

2 Work the trachea and larynx by applying pressure along the edge of the big toe joint, to stimulate these organs to clear and heal.

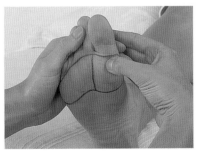

4 Work the thyroid helper area in the section of the chest under the big toe. Finish by working the entire chest area for a boost to the respiratory system.

colour meditation

Tap into the power of the mind to bring healing and wellbeing to the body. Use meditation and creative visualization to encourage a speedy recovery from colds and other common complaints.

This healing meditation is best done sitting or lying down somewhere warm and quiet where you will not be disturbed for around 15–20 minutes. The meditation can be practised at any time of the day, or last thing at night to promote a restful sleep.

healing with colour

Begin by imagining a healing glow of coloured light surrounding your body. Let that colour become stronger and then as you breathe in, imagine it flowing into the top of your head. As you continue to relax, let the coloured light begin to suffuse all areas of your body, starting with the head, face, neck and shoulders, and travel down, penetrating all the muscles and organs. Fill up every part of your body until it is completely suffused with a warm, healing light.

As you relax, bring your attention to the head, throat and chest area, or any other area of the body you feel drawn to. Draw in more warmth and colour on the in-breath and send it to this area. Imagine it giving power, helping to strengthen the cells and

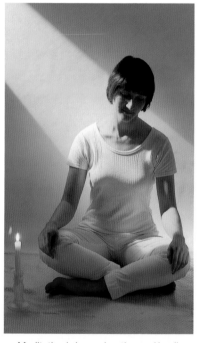

▲ *Meditation brings relaxation and healing.*

fight off germs. Imagine your body free of aches and pains and any illness.

When you feel the healing is complete, allow the light to disperse, letting it go with each exhalation. Gently stretch your body as you return to the everyday world.

amethyst healing

Crystals and stones are used in healing to magnify and transform energy. Amethyst quartz is one of the most useful healing stones. Its cleansing and balancing properties can be used to treat a cold.

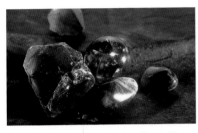

◀ *Amethyst quartz is one of the most versatile healing stones.*

Many healers believe that illness originates in the body's subtle energy system of chakras and auras. Crystals can be used to help realign these energies and bring about healing.

For a cold that lingers on and won't seem to shift, you could try treating it on another level, using amethyst points to rebalance and repair any "holes" in the aura.

crystal cold cure

Make sure you can lie somewhere warm and quiet for 20–30 minutes, where you won't be disturbed. You may like to play a piece of soothing music during the relaxation. Take eight amethysts of roughly equal size, and space them out evenly around the body. If the stones are faceted, place them so that the points are facing inwards; this will focus the healing energy towards the body. Now lie back and relax as the stones realign your aura.

▼ *Amethyst balances and quietens the mind.*

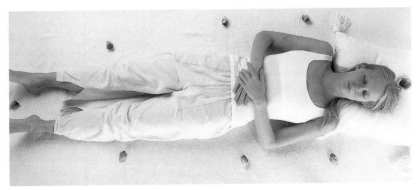

99 go to bed

Sleep is probably one of the greatest natural healers of all. Sometimes the body just needs a chance to rest and recuperate from the stresses and strains of daily life.

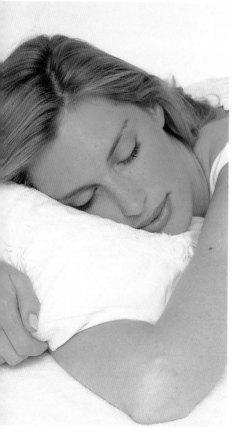

When you have a cold or flu, make sure you have plenty of rest and sleep – this alone will go a long way towards a quick recovery. Always make sure you sleep in a well-ventilated room. It is better to put an extra blanket on the bed and sleep with the window slightly open than to spend the night in a stuffy, overheated room.

▼ *A lavender sachet beside the bed may help to induce sleep.*

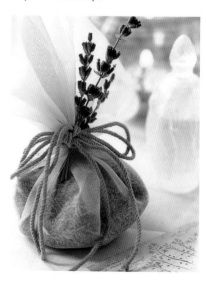

▲ *One of the best cures for a cold is to make yourself a herb or spice tea and go straight to bed.*

Try resting your head on a

sleep pillow

filled with mild sedative

herbs and flowers such as

hops or

lavender.

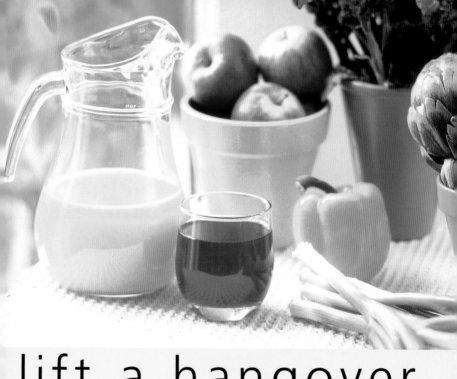

lift a hangover

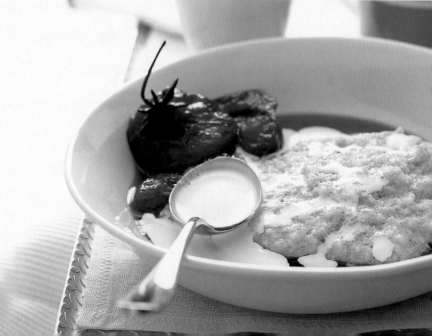

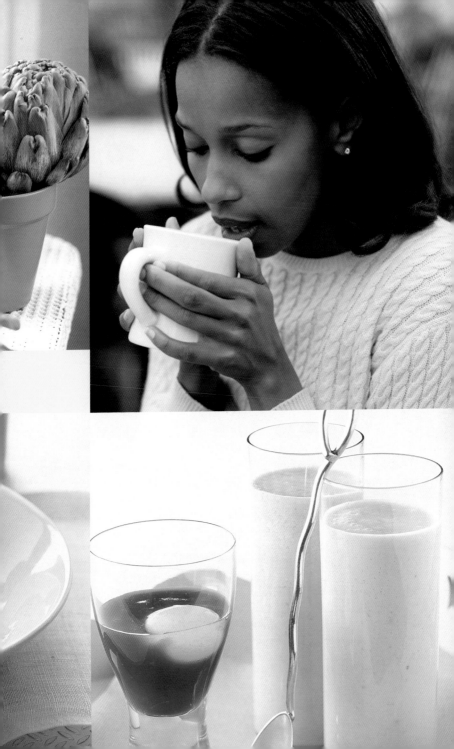

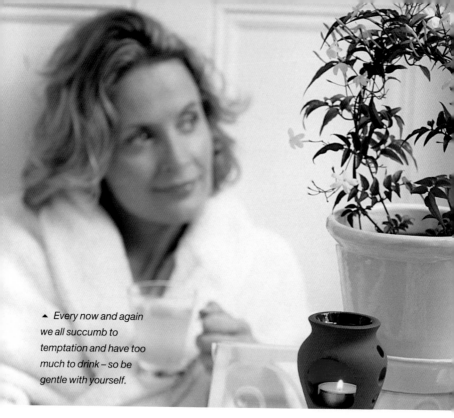

▲ *Every now and again we all succumb to temptation and have too much to drink – so be gentle with yourself.*

how to cure a hangover

Dog breath, a throbbing head, churning stomach and a mouth like the inside of a birdcage. If these nasty symptoms sound horribly familiar then there is every chance that you are one of the countless millions of people who knows exactly what it feels like to suffer from a hangover. According to the dictionary, a hangover may be defined as the unpleasant effects resulting from excessive alcohol consumption. It literally means a remnant from the past (a hang-over) – or in other words, it is the morning after the night before.

So why exactly do you feel quite so ghastly? Put simply, alcohol is a drug with fairly brutal side effects. When consumed in moderate amounts, your body can produce enough enzymes to metabolize the toxins from the alcohol and you don't notice any adverse reactions. But when your level of alcohol consumption exceeds your body's ability to cope, you have all the nasty symptoms of a classic hangover. These include headaches, nausea, diarrhoea, dehydration and dizziness, together with irritability, fatigue and general aches and pains. They are the telltale signs that your body is struggling to deal with toxic overload and are a mild and temporary version of what drug addicts suffer when they experience withdrawal symptoms. A hangover is nature's way of telling you that you have been overdoing it.

congenial congeners

The excess toxins in your system seem to come from two sources. Some are present in the alcoholic drink itself, while others get created as a metabolic by-product of the liver. During the fermentation process of certain fruits or grains, the chemical compound ethanol (alcohol) is produced and this is what is responsible for a drink's intoxicating effect. At the same time, toxic by-products of the fermentation process are also created. Known as 'congeners', these chemical impurities contribute to each drink's characteristic taste, colour and aroma, and are what the liver must process. Hence it is a good idea to avoid mixing your drinks as this means the body has to work even harder in its clean-up operations. As a rule, clear wines and spirits such as vodka, gin or white wine contain fewer congeners than dark, full-bodied alcoholic drinks such as red wine, brandy or bourbon. Although congeners do not cause drunkenness, they do seem to contribute to how ill you feel afterwards. This may help to explain why the effect of drinking lighter coloured liquors seems to be slightly less devastating than drinking dark ones, an idea supported by medical research.

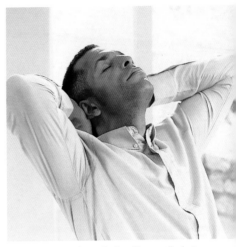

▲ The next day it can be hard to recall what was so wonderful about the night before.

feeling unwell

When the alcohol enters your bloodstream, your liver starts to produce an enzyme called 'alcohol dehydrogenase' (ADH) to break it down. Habitual drinkers have built up higher levels of ADH, which helps to explain their increased tolerance to alcohol. There is also some research to suggest that men tend to produce more of this enzyme than women and are thus able to 'hold' their drink better. As the liver gets to work, the enzymes also produce acetaldehyde, a highly toxic substance that can make you feel very unwell.

As alcohol is a diuretic, your kidneys are geared into action to pass more water than usual. It is also the body's way of trying to eliminate toxins as speedily as possible. If you do not compensate with extra liquid (non-alcoholic of course), then this impacts on the rest of the body as

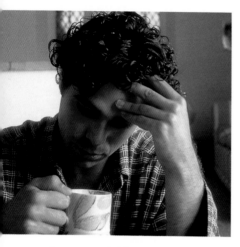

◄ *A thumping headache is a common hangover symptom. This is partly the result of being dehydrated.*

you know drinking too much is bad for you, and however many times you've sworn 'never again', there's every chance that sooner or later you're going to overdo it and once more seek solace in your favourite hangover remedy.

natural treatments

Before turning to the painkillers and pumping more drugs into your system, there are ways of treating a hangover that can support your body's natural processes rather than simply obliterating the pain. Whether you are suffering a crashing headache, a queasy tummy, or general debility, this section is packed with a variety of drug-free treatments to help alleviate some of the symptoms of a hangover. It is hoped that you will find the suggestions fun as well as useful and discover a variety of different treatments that will work for you.

whatever fluid is available is redistributed, leading to dehydration – with even your brain becoming dry and 'pickled'. This loss of body fluids is considered to be one of the major causes of hangover symptoms and, of course, is exacerbated by vomiting and diarrhoea. Although it may feel awful, vomiting and/or diarrhoea is actually a healthy response since it is the body's way of throwing out the poisons that are flooding your system.

never say never again

Excess drinking on a regular basis puts a great strain on your body. It is an addictive, expensive habit that has many unpleasant and harmful side effects. Too much alcohol depletes the body of essential vitamins and minerals and adversely affects blood sugar levels. High blood pressure, liver damage, digestive disorders, impaired mental functioning, as well as unhealthy, tired-looking skin are just some of the consequences of long-term alcohol abuse. Yet although

GOLDEN RULES

Before going out on the town, remember the following and you may save yourself an awful hangover experience.

- never drink on an empty stomach.
- eat absorbent 'bulky' foods rather than crisps, sticks of celery or nuts.
- don't mix your drinks.
- alternate each alcoholic drink with a non-alcoholic one.

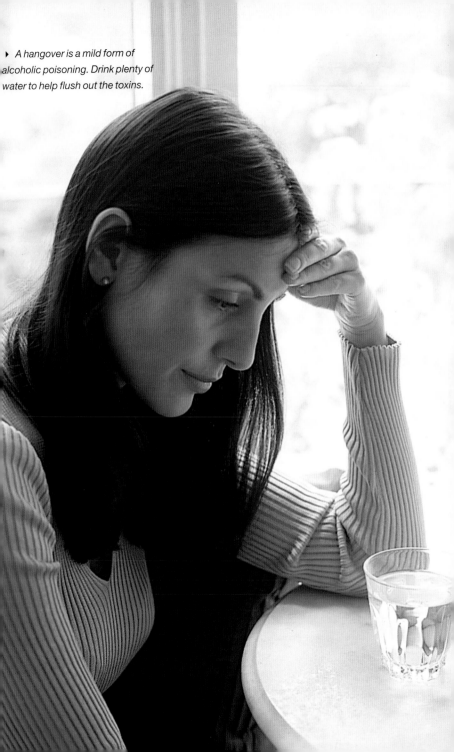

▸ *A hangover is a mild form of alcoholic poisoning. Drink plenty of water to help flush out the toxins.*

hangover treatments

The quest for the perfect hangover cure is rather like the search for the Holy Grail. It has enduring fascination yet somehow remains tantalizingly out of reach. After centuries of ingenious suggestions it is probably fairly safe to conclude that there is no single perfect cure for a hangover – other than letting nature take its course. But there are steps you can take to help nature do its work and support a speedy recovery.

The pages that follow present 50 tried and tested safe and natural treatments. Some of these are aimed at quick-fix solutions while others are targeted at improving your body's defences and strengthening resistance to hangover symptoms. They are drawn from a variety of approaches to natural healthcare and include holistic therapies such as homeopathy, reflexology, aromatherapy and colour healing, as well as diet and nutrition where a wide variety of healing foods and drinks as well as herbs and vitamins are included.

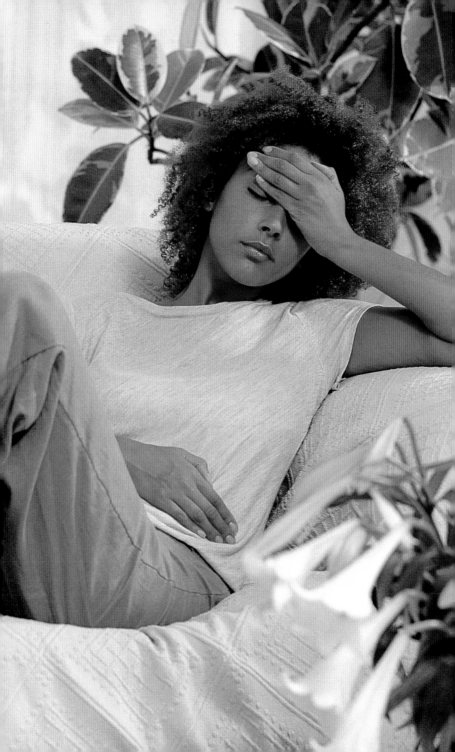

101

fortifying echinacea

Echinacea is a traditional Native American medicine. Taken regularly, the plant's healing powers will help the body overcome the negative effects of over-indulgence in alcohol.

In the 1950s Ben Black Elk, a Sioux from South Dakota, gave a parting gift to the visiting Swiss 'nature' doctor Alfred Vogel. This gift was a handful of seeds from the coneflower (*Echinacea purpurea*) plant, the most powerful remedy Black Elk knew. Nowadays, echinacea is widely cultivated for its amazing healing properties. Although the plant has a particularly strong affinity with the respiratory tract, it is also a powerful blood cleanser and immunity booster.

building defences

Echinacea may not ease your hangover headache, but taken regularly it will help build and strengthen your immune system, keep your system clean and assist a speedy recovery when you do get sick – whether from illness or the effects of alcohol poisoning. During the party season when late nights, too much booze and poor eating habits are guaranteed to take their toll, using echinacea will help build your body's defences so you can party until you drop.

Echinacea is prepared as a herbal remedy from the plant's roots and

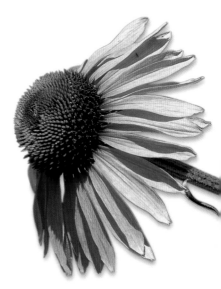

▲ *Echinacea is a powerful immunity booster. Take it regularly as a preventative measure to strengthen your system.*

leaves, although the best remedies are allegedly those that are made using the entire plant. It is available in tincture or tablet form from good health stores and pharmacies. As a preventative measure, you could take 2.5ml (½ tsp) tincture in a little water or juice once a day, or one 500mg capsule twice a day.

102 ginseng boost

In Chinese medicine, ginseng is the number one tonic and healer. For centuries in the East, top grade roots have been valued more highly than gold and imbued with almost magical properties.

In parts of Asia, ginseng plants up to 200 years old can still be found. It is believed that those lucky enough to acquire such plants can live to a ripe old age, as ginseng is said to increase longevity. Ginseng has a strengthening effect on the nervous system and improves tolerance to stress. It also aids recovery from illness, fights fatigue and boosts alertness. Although there are many varieties of ginseng, the Korean variety (*panax ginseng*) is believed to be the most powerful. Siberian ginseng (*eleutherococcus*) has a similar action and is particularly helpful for combating fatigue.

body balancer
Ginseng is a useful hangover remedy because it works to bring the body back into balance. It contains vitamins, minerals and amino acids, and helps to balance blood sugar levels in the body. Ginseng helps to protect and strengthen the liver against toxic overload. It is also a powerful immune system booster and helps combat the effects of stress. All very important if you want to avoid feeling lousy.

Although it is possible to make ginseng tea by boiling up the powdered root, most people find it more convenient to take regular supplements in tablet form, widely available in good health stores and pharmacies. Take up to two 600mg tablets daily, or as directed.

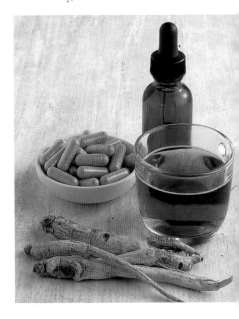

▸ *Ginseng root may be boiled up in a little water to make a tea or else it is available as a tincture or as capsules.*

103 milk thistle detox

In herbal medicine, milk thistle has a long tradition of use. It is the herbal remedy most commonly used for healing and protecting the liver and its many metabolic activities.

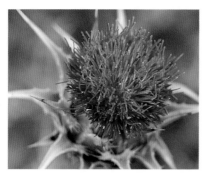

▲ Milk thistle is a powerful liver protector.

Native to the Mediterranean regions, this silvery-edged thorny leaved plant thrives in humid, salty sea air and stony soil where it can grow up to 2m (6ft) high. Silymarin, the active component of milk thistle (*Silybum marianum*), is found in the plant's seeds and it is this substance that is so effective in protecting the liver.

liver reviver

Studies have shown that silymarin can prevent severe liver damage after ingesting highly toxic compounds, while it has also been used successfully to treat hepatitis and liver cirrhosis. Milk thistle can help to regenerate a damaged liver and stimulate the production of healthy new cells; it also has a cleansing and purifying effect and encourages the liver to work more efficiently.

It is these therapeutic actions that make milk thistle such a valuable hangover remedy, as it is the liver that has to cope with all the nasty effects caused by alcoholic excess. When you have a busy social time ahead, try taking a four-week preventative course. A suggested dose would be one 500mg capsule three times a day. Or take one 500mg capsule three times a day as a first-aid measure when you have a hangover. Milk thistle is also available in tincture form.

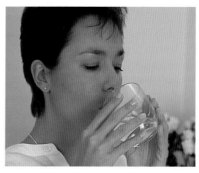

▲ A milk thistle capsule taken with a glass of water should help a hangover.

cleansing artichokes

Most of us are familiar with globe artichokes as a rather exotic looking vegetable. Yet this tasty plant also has an important reputation in herbal medicine for treating liver disorders.

Like milk thistle, the artichoke (*Cynara scolymus*) plant is native to the Mediterranean region. Similarly, it is also recognized as a valuable liver tonic. The green parts of the plant contain the compound cynaropicrin, which is what gives the vegetable its characteristic aroma and bitter taste. This bitterness stimulates liver and gall-bladder function, making the artichoke useful for the treatment of gall-bladder problems and digestive disorders. The plant's leaves also contain cynarin, another valuable substance that acts on the liver in a similar way to silymarin, found in milk thistle. In addition, artichokes are rich in antioxidants.

liver cleanser

Taking artichoke will help protect your liver against toxins and minimize the damage caused by drinking alcohol. It will also encourage a speedier clean-up operation. Like most herbal remedies, the plant is commercially available in tincture or capsule form, which makes it easy to use. To treat a hangover, take one 500mg capsule three times a day. Alternatively try a short course to help your liver detox, taking one 500mg capsule three times a day for four weeks. Eating the fresh vegetable is also helpful.

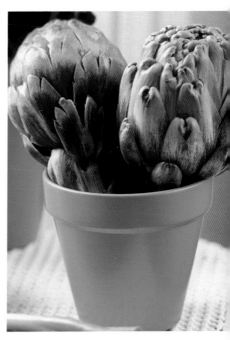

▶ *Artichokes have a distinctive, bitter taste that stimulates liver function. The herbal remedy is a good detoxifier.*

105 soothing slippery elm

Best known as a herb for treating stomach complaints, slippery elm's soothing action is wonderful for an overwrought digestive system. It should help to settle your upset stomach.

The slippery elm (*Ulmus rubra*) tree is native to Canada and the United States. It is the tree's inner bark that is used in herbal medicine. The trees must be at least ten years old and during the spring, their bark is collected, dried and then powdered. Slippery elm bark contains a viscous solution (mucilage) which gives rise to its 'slippery' taste and texture – and also the tree's name. This mucilage has a soothing action in the gut, reducing inflammation and calming spasms, making it a useful herbal remedy for a wide range of digestive disorders, including acid indigestion, diarrhoea and gastroenteritis.

speedy stomach settler
Slippery elm is available in good health stores and pharmacies and is usually sold in either powder, capsule or tablet form. For instant relief from an upset stomach, make yourself a nourishing – if slimy – drink from the powder. Mix a little powder to a paste with cold water and then top up with hot water, using a ratio of 1 part powder to 8 parts water, or follow the instructions on the jar. If you prefer, substitute the hot water with hot milk, particularly if it's last thing at night, as this may help you sleep. If you feel too sick to stomach it, then take your slippery elm in tablet or capsule form and this should help settle your heaving insides. A 400mg dose should be sufficient, followed by two 200mg doses at three-hourly intervals if needed.

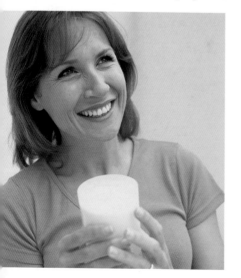

◀ *Slippery elm is not to everyone's taste but it is a good stomach soother.*

106 stomach settler

Fiery ginger and aromatic cloves are two of the best natural remedies for alleviating digestive upsets such as nausea , vomiting and flatulence. Ginger is also an excellent digestive tonic.

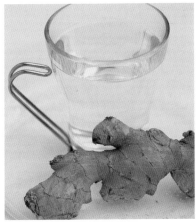

▲ A glass of fresh ginger tea will help to settle your stomach and alleviate nausea.

Apart from its versatility as a culinary spice, ginger is probably best known as an antidote to nausea and vomiting, whether this is caused by motion sickness, by morning sickness during pregnancy, or by sickness caused by over-indulgence. There is plenty of evidence to point to the effectiveness of root ginger in this area: in medical trials, for instance, the spice has been found to be more effective than conventional medicines at relieving post-operative nausea.

Although less well known, cloves have similar restorative properties to ginger. They are generally used to assist the action of other medicines rather than on their own.

sickness suppressor

Ginger helps to settle the stomach and ease abdominal pain, distension and flatulent indigestion as well as relaxing muscular spasm. It is also a powerful antioxidant, inhibiting free radicals in the body and stimulating the speedy removal of toxins. It is to all these properties that ginger owes its reputation as a good hangover cure.

There are a variety of ways to take ginger. The crystallized root can be chewed as a sweet, the powdered root taken in capsule form, or the fresh root boiled to make a drink. It is also available in tincture form. Add 3–4 drops to a glass of water and sip at intervals. (Note: the tincture should not be confused with ginger essential oil, which should not be ingested.)

To make a clove infusion steep ½–1oz cloves in freshly boiled water for 5–10 minutes. Alternatively, add a little clove powder to a ginger tea.

natural tonics

One of nature's most valuable plants, evening primrose is best known for its oil. This contains many nourishing properties and is said to counter the effects of alcoholic poisoning.

The fragrant yellow flowers of the evening primrose plant (*Oenothera biennis*) open at dusk, attracting the night-flying insects that pollinate them. The plant was known to the Ancient Greeks, and the flower's generic name is derived from two Greek words: 'oinos' meaning wine, and 'thera' meaning hunt. This refers to the plant's reputation to stimulate a desire for wine and/or to dispel the effects of over-indulgence. You can only judge for yourself how far this is true, but a great deal of research has been made into the medicinal effects of evening primrose oil, which is derived from the plant's seeds.

system replenisher

Evening primrose oil is an excellent source of Omega 6 fatty acids, which are vital for the healthy functioning of the immune, nervous and hormonal systems. Evening primrose oil also contains gamma linolenic acid (GLA), a precursor of prostaglandin E1 – a mood enhancer. Unfortunately alcoholic binges upset the healthy functioning of the body's systems and this enhancer can be destroyed.

Taking evening primrose oil can help to realign metabolic disturbances after drinking. Studies have also shown that it can help with alcohol withdrawal symptoms and alcoholic depression, as well as helping the liver to regenerate. The most convenient way of taking evening primrose oil is in capsules, widely available in health stores and pharmacies. For a hangover take 3–5 1,000mg capsules. Evening primrose is sometimes blended with starflower oil, which works in a similar way.

▲ *Evening primrose oil can help with the symptoms of alcohol withdrawal.*

108 top up on vitamin C

Drinking alcohol, along with smoking and stress, rapidly uses up vitamin C. As this vitamin is crucial to maintaining a healthy immune system it is important to keep levels topped up.

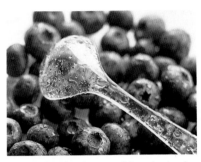

▲ Fresh blueberries are a rich and natural source of vitamin C.

Vitamin C is water-soluble and any excess is excreted when you urinate. As your body is unable to store or produce this vitamin, it relies on you having an adequate daily intake.

Normally, vitamin C is excreted in two to three hours, but because alcohol is a diuretic, elimination is faster and your body's vitamin C requirement dramatically increases. The situation is compounded by smoking, as each cigarette destroys 25mg of vitamin C. To help redress the balance, especially if you have been in a smoky environment, a therapeutic dose of 1,000mg should help you on the way to recovery. This dose can be repeated every two to three hours as needed. If you are taking ginseng, leave a three-hour gap before or after taking vitamin C.

vitamin C sources

Many people supplement their diet with vitamin pills or powders, but the best source of vitamin C is fresh fruit. Citrus fruits, rosehips, blackcurrants, berries and broccoli are especially rich in this vitamin, although it is also found in all other fresh fruit and vegetables. A good way of taking in a large dose is to drink fruit juices, either shop-bought or home-pressed. The liquid in fruit and juices will also help replenish the body's water levels.

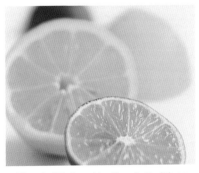

▲ Vitamin C is found in citrus fruits. It is an immunity booster and antioxidant.

vitamin B1

The B vitamins are synergistic, which means they work best when taken together as a B-complex. It is vitamin B1, however, that offers most protection against alcoholic excess.

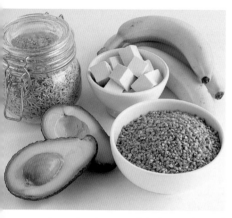

▲ Avocados, bananas, tofu, brown rice and most wholegrains are all high in B vitamins.

There are more than ten members of the vitamin B group and they play an essential role in more than 60 metabolic reactions. They are particularly involved in energy production and in the manufacture of red blood cells but are probably most well known for their effect on the nervous system.

vitamin B sources

As a rule, B vitamins are found more abundantly in vegetables rather than fruit, although avocados and bananas are high in B vitamins. Other good natural sources include wheat bran, yeast, fish, liver, eggs, milk and cheese.

Known as the 'feel good' vitamin, B1 (thiamine) has a beneficial effect on mood and general well-being, helping you feel calm, clear-headed and energetic. Low levels of thiamine are associated with lack of self-confidence and depression. Caffeine, alcohol, stress and smoking are all enemies of B1 and it may come as little surprise to find that B1 deficiency is very common. However, of all the B vitamins, it is B1 that seems to offer the most protection against a hangover and is even reputed to decrease your taste for alcohol. It is found in all plant and animal foods, but especially rich sources are brown rice, wholegrains, seafood and legumes.

To help prevent a hangover, take one high-strength B-complex tablet before drinking, one during drinking and one before you go to bed. To ease the symptoms of a hangover, take a high-strength B-complex together with a multi-vitamin and mineral tablet and repeat six hours later.

110 water, water, water

Dehydration is one of the main reasons for feeling hung over. While you are enjoying alcoholic beverages your body is actually losing fluids. Drinking water is a top cure.

The importance of drinking water cannot be stressed enough. Your body is largely made up of this vital, life-giving element and it covers more than two-thirds of the earth's surface. It is not for nothing that it is called the elixir of life.

keep topping up

To stop yourself feeling like death the morning after, make sure you drink plenty of water before you go out drinking, plenty more while you are indulging, a large glass of the stuff before you go to bed, and another large glass when you wake up. In any case health experts recommend that you should be drinking at least 1.5 litres/2½ pints/6¼ cups a day to keep you in tip-top condition – and that is before a drop of alcohol has passed your lips.

Drinking plenty of water before, during and after a drinking session will help your body in two main ways. Alcohol is a diuretic and dehydrates your body fairly dramatically. Drinking plenty of water helps to hydrate your body in preparation for the huge fluid loss caused by the booze. Secondly, it will help flush out the evil toxins that are making you feel so dreadful. Don't worry if you need to urinate more than normal – it's a small price to pay given the circumstances.

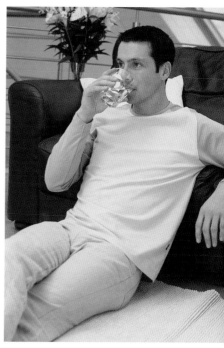

▲ *Drinking plenty of water is one of the easiest ways to treat a hangover.*

111

spicy orange zinger

When you feel like crawling under a stone to die, zing is probably the last thing on your mind. Yet this spicy fruit cocktail can soon change that.

Fresh fruit juices can send a hangover on its way. Like water, juices help to flush your system of toxins and rehydrate your body, which will hopefully quieten that loud, thumping headache and get rid of that awful giddy feeling.

ancient remedy

The following drink combines fresh fruit juices with spices and is based on a traditional Ayurvedic remedy. Originating in India, Ayurveda is one of the oldest healthcare systems in the world and makes great use of nutritious foods and drinks in its treatments. Spices in particular are very important, as it is not just their taste that counts, but each has unique healing properties. To make enough for one serving, you will need the juice of 2–3 freshly squeezed large oranges, plus 10ml/2 tsp fresh lime juice and a pinch of cumin. Give the ingredients a good stir to mix well and serve immediately as fresh juices lose their potency if they are left standing around for too long.

The drink should not only taste delightful to your jaded taste buds but it is also packed with nutrients. Both oranges and limes of course are high in vitamin C and will give your immune system a much-needed boost. In Ayurvedic medicine, cumin is seen to have a cooling effect on the body and is therefore helpful in disorders associated with excess heat. After over-indulging, acid indigestion and wind are just some of the signs of an inflamed digestive system. So drink up and restore your body to balance as quickly and painlessly as possible.

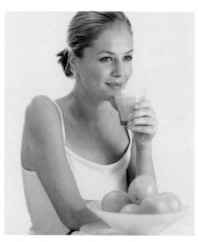

▲ *Freshly squeezed orange, lime and cumin is an Ayurvedic hangover remedy.*

112 virgin bloody mary

The reason you feel so awful is because your body is going through mild withdrawal symptoms from an alcohol overdose. Try this if you feel tempted by a curative top-up.

A Bloody Mary is a vodka and tomato juice cocktail and is probably one of the most infamous hangover cures of all. It is based on the 'hair of the dog' principle, which argues that since your hangover is caused by withdrawal symptoms, if you give yourself a top-up with more alcohol, your ghastly symptoms will subside and you will soon feel better. Ironically there is some truth in this. The effects, however, are only temporary and eventually you will have to sober up and face the loud, discordant music going on inside your skull. In any case you probably know deep down that it's not really a good idea to succumb to temptation. It will only mask your symptoms temporarily and if it became a habit, it could lead to alcohol abuse and a serious drinking problem.

healthy 'hair of the dog'

If all this sounds boringly sensible, then trick yourself with the next best thing. This Virgin Bloody Mary looks and almost tastes the same as the genuine article but it won't cause you any harm. In fact it is more than likely

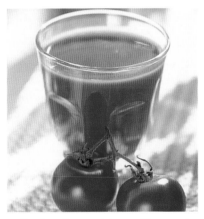

▲ Raw tomatoes contain over 90 per cent water and are said to be good for reducing liver inflammation.

to do you some good – tomatoes are alkali forming, and help to reduce stomach acidity. To make one serving you will need 300ml/½ pint/1¼ cups fresh or bottled tomato juice, juice of ½ lemon, Tabasco sauce, Worcestershire sauce, salt and pepper. Mix the tomato and lemon juice together and season to suit your taste with the rest of the ingredients. Finally, add a handful of ice for that wonderful clinking sound, put your feet up and sip through a long straw.

113 blackcurrant & cranberry breeze

When you're out on a drinking spree, your kidneys are working extra hard to flush the fluids from your system. Why not give them a helping hand with this tasty tonic?

Blackcurrants and cranberries each deserve their well-earned reputation as 'super foods'. Both fruits have a high vitamin C content and are rich in nutrients and healing properties. This makes their juice a wonderful tonic for a body under stress – an apt description for your poor hungover system.

Blackcurrants have a blood cleansing and purifying action, while a compound in their purple-black skin is a powerful anti-inflammatory.

This is what makes blackcurrants such a good sore throat remedy, but the same soothing properties can be put to good use to ease acid indigestion, relax intestinal spasms and stem diarrhoea. Cranberries on the other hand, with their antibacterial and strengthening properties, have a specific affinity with the kidneys and urinary tract. They have a tart, bitter taste and so work well when mixed with sweeter fruits like blackcurrants.

refresher juice

To make enough for one serving you will need 75g/3oz blackcurrants and 150g/5oz cranberries. You will also need a juicing machine. Remove the stalks from the blackcurrants and rinse the currants and the cranberries. Do not chop or peel. Put the fruit through the juicer and add a little honey to taste. If fresh fruits are not available, or you simply can't be bothered, then use ready-made juices instead. Cranberry is available in most supermarkets, while blackcurrant is sold in all good health stores. Make sure it is blackcurrant juice rather than a cordial.

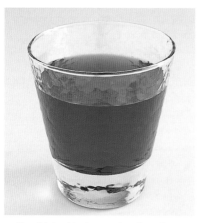

▲ Combining blackcurrant and cranberry juice makes a tasty, healing tonic which is especially beneficial for your kidneys.

114 banana smoothie

Potassium is one of the body's most important minerals and is seriously depleted through alcoholic excess. Bananas are one of the best sources of potassium.

Potassium is crucial for body functioning. It maintains the water balance within your body's cells and stabilizes their internal structure. It also plays a central role in energy production and helps to conduct nerve impulses through the body. When your body loses fluids, whether through sweating, vomiting, diarrhoea, or from diuretics, then potassium is leached away. Symptoms of potassium deficiency include muscular weakness, muscle pains and overwhelming fatigue, which are all common hangover symptoms.

energy boosting bananas
Bananas are packed with potassium and are an instant energy food. They also contain zinc, iron, and vitamins C and B6. Natural antacids, bananas can also restore an angry digestive system to normal functioning. For maximum benefit, bananas should be eaten ripe; they are less effective when they are still green around the tips. Avoid bruised or greyish bananas, but opt for plump fruit with a good colour.

For an instant energy-boosting drink that will also soothe your weary system this banana smoothie should do the trick. This delicious thick and fruity drink is mixed with yogurt and/or milk.

To make enough for one serving you will need 1 good-sized ripe banana, 120ml/4fl oz/½ cup skimmed milk and 50ml/2fl oz/¼ cup natural live yogurt. Peel the banana and put all the ingredients into a blender and blend until smooth. Add more milk if you like a runnier consistency and serve chilled or on ice.

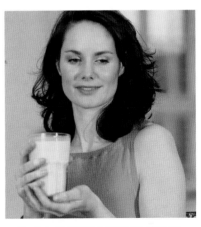

▲ *For instant energy, a nourishing banana smoothie will soon put the bounce back in your step.*

115 green energy

Fresh juices have remarkable cleansing and restorative powers. Green veggie juices in particular are great for detoxing the body's systems and strengthening the liver.

A detox programme is the classical treatment for weaning addicts off alcohol and drugs. Although no one is suggesting that you are alcohol dependent, a detox remains one of the best natural treatments for a hangover. For a simple detox, drinking fresh vegetable juice is one of the simplest and most effective cures. Vegetable juices have a much milder action in the body than fruit juices and are also excellent restoratives and should soon put you back on your feet.

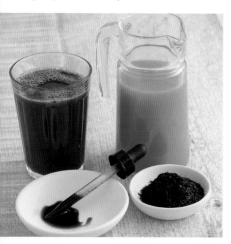

▲ Dark green vegetable juices are potent detoxifiers and energy boosters.

Chlorophyll is the 'green blood' of plants that enables them to harvest the sun's life-giving energy. It has potent cleansing properties and is what makes green vegetables so helpful in a detox. As a rule, the darker green the vegetable, the more potent its potential detoxing and curative powers. Dark green vegetables are also rich in B vitamins and minerals.

detox veggie juice
This 'green energy' juice is made from spinach and celery, although you could substitute watercress, curly kale or cabbage for the spinach if you prefer. Celery is included for its high water content and its toning effect on the kidneys. According to traditional herbal medicine it also calms the nerves. To make enough for one serving you will need 2 sticks of celery and a large handful of spinach leaves. Wash the veggies and put them in a juice extractor. If you wish, you could mix with a little fresh carrot juice for flavour. Drink up immediately, as the juice will lose its potency if it is left standing around.

116 prairie oyster

The desire for a hangover cure has led to many strange experimental remedies. Raw eels, soused herrings and raw eggs have all been popular. A prairie oyster is a type of egg nog.

In the Middle Ages, hangover sufferers swore by a mixture that included raw eel, while in Holland a whole soused herring slipped down the back of the throat is meant to work wonders. It's difficult to know on what basis some of these cures are founded, suffice to say that if you can swallow it down without throwing it up then you must be on the way to a speedy recovery – or else you're still too drunk to notice!

eggy hangover cure

A prairie oyster is based on the 'hair of the dog that bit me' premise and uses a vodka or brandy base. It is equally effective without the alcohol as it is the raw egg that does the trick. Maybe this is because eggs contain cysteine, which is said to clean up destructive chemicals that build up in the liver while metabolizing excess alcohol.

To make a prairie oyster mix 25ml/ 1½ tbsp apple cider vinegar, 25ml/ 1½ tbsp Worcestershire sauce, 5ml/ 1 tsp tomato ketchup, 5ml/1 tsp Angostura bitters and a dash of Tabasco in a tumbler. If you really want to go for the full hair of the dog, then add 25ml/1½ tbsp of either brandy or vodka, but this is strictly optional. Finally, drop in a raw egg yolk and knock it back without breaking the yolk. Make sure that the bathroom is within striking distance!

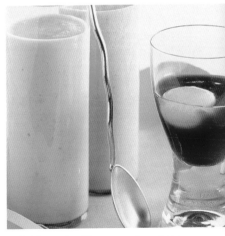

▲ *Drinks made with raw eggs have been popular hangover cures for centuries.*

> **CAUTIONS**
> • Children, pregnant women and the elderly should avoid eating raw eggs.
>
> • Free-range organic eggs are the safest choice when using them raw.

117 peppermint tea

Herbal teas are excellent natural hangover remedies. Peppermint is a firm favourite as it is healing for an upset digestive system and makes a refreshing start to the day.

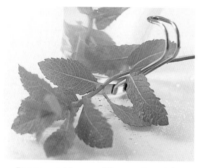

▲ *Peppermint is one of the most useful and effective herbal hangover remedies.*

If you feel tempted to sober up with a black coffee, think again. Coffee will dehydrate and irritate your system still further, and contrary to popular opinion, it will do nothing for your hangover – except make you feel more awake perhaps. For a therapeutic wake-up call, peppermint tea is a much better way to stimulate your groggy self into action.

reviving peppermint

Peppermint (*Mentha* X *piperita*) has always been valued for its stimulating, refreshing effects. Centuries ago, the Roman historian, Pliny (AD23–79) stated: 'the very smell of mint restores and revives the spirits just as its taste excites the appetite'. It is the volatile oil in the plant's leaves that creates peppermint's distinctive aroma and gives it its therapeutic powers. This essential oil should not be ingested directly, but the plant's fresh or dried leaves may be infused in hot water and made into tea.

Peppermint is a top herbal remedy for nausea and indigestion. When taken internally, it brings relief for conditions associated with pain and spasm, including stomach ache, wind, heart burn, indigestion, hiccups and vomiting. Peppermint helps to protect the gut lining from irritation and infection, and relieves griping pains during diarrhoea. It also has a cleansing and detoxing effect on the liver.

minty brew

For a refreshing peppermint tea, use 5ml/1 tsp dried peppermint leaves or 10ml/2 tsp fresh herbs per 250ml/8fl oz/1 cup of near-boiling water. Steep the herbs in the water for 5–10 minutes, then drain off the liquid into a cup and drink while hot. If you need a sweetener, stir in a little honey.

118

lemon, lime & ginger toddy

Like lemons, limes are high in vitamin C as well as B vitamins. Their unique citrus flavours combine with ginger in this hot toddy that will ease a horrible hangover.

We generally think of lemons and limes as being very acidic and may conclude that they are best avoided when suffering from an upset stomach. However, the fruits' acidic properties are metabolized during digestion to produce potassium carbonate, which actually helps neutralize excess acid in the body. Furthermore, lemon juice has a protective action on the membranous lining of the digestive tract, making it useful to help prevent stomach upsets.

Both lemons and limes are also a tonic for the liver and pancreas. They have a cleansing and purifying action that helps to remove toxic wastes and impurities and restore the body to a state of homeostasis (balance). Their taste and healing properties are complemented by ginger, which in itself is an excellent remedy for nausea and stomach upsets.

comforting hot toddy

To make a lemon, lime and ginger toddy, take a 115g/4oz piece of washed fresh root ginger and slice it into 600ml/1 pint/2½ cups water. Bring the water to the boil, cover and gently simmer the root for 15–20 minutes. Meanwhile squeeze 1 medium-sized lemon and 1 lime and put the juice to one side. When the ginger has finished cooking, remove it from the heat and strain the liquid into a cup. Allow it to cool slightly before adding the citrus juices. Sweeten with honey to taste, go back to bed and sip slowly.

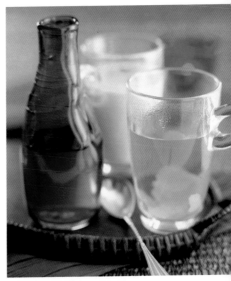

▲ A hot toddy made with lemon, lime and ginger is an excellent restorative.

119

dandelion & marshmallow brew

Although dandelion is infamous as a weed, it is important in herbal medicine because of its detoxifying, bitter properties. Combine it with marshmallow for a potent hangover drink.

Both the leaves and root of the unassuming dandelion plant (*Taraxacum officinale*) have a therapeutic action on the kidneys and liver. Dandelion's edible and bitter leaves are a powerful diuretic, but unlike most conventional diuretics that leach the body of potassium, they actually contain high levels of the mineral. This creates an ideal balance, helping the kidneys flush out toxins on the one hand, while simultaneously keeping the body's potassium levels high. Dandelion root is also a very effective detoxifying herb. Although its main area of action is on the liver and gall-bladder, it also has a stimulating effect on the kidneys and helps the body to excrete toxins via the urine.

Known as the flower of softness, the high mucilage content of marshmallow (*Althaea officinalis*) makes it useful whenever a soothing effect is needed. Marshmallow root is used primarily for stomach problems and inflammations of the digestive tract. It counters excess stomach acid and soothes an irritable bowel.

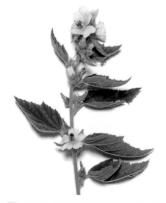

▲ The root of the marshmallow plant is often used to settle the stomach.

stomach settling brew

A dandelion and marshmallow brew is a fantastic detoxing hangover cure that is kind to your insides. To make a brew, add 10g/¼oz each of dried dandelion and marshmallow root to 600ml/1 pint/2½ cups water and simmer for 10 minutes. When the roots have softened add 5g/⅛oz each of dried dandelion and marshmallow leaves to the hot water, cover and leave to infuse for a further 5 minutes. If using fresh herbs, double the quantities. Strain off the liquid and drink while still warm.

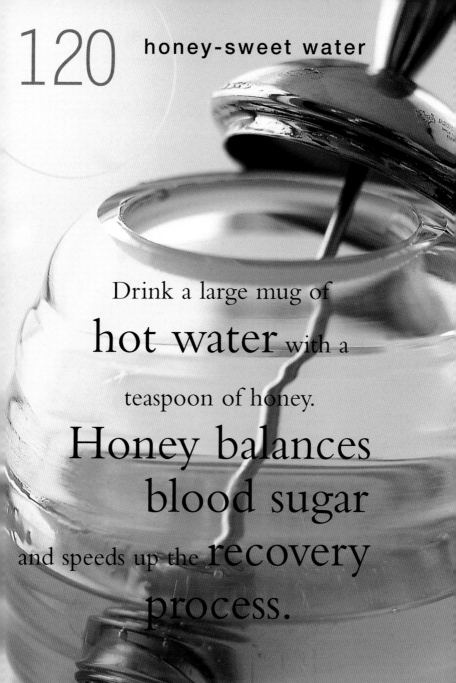

Drink a large mug of
hot water with a
teaspoon of honey.
Honey balances
blood sugar
and speeds up the recovery
process.

121 green tea

It's official – green tea is not only a refreshing drink, but it's also good for you. It has many health-giving properties and is a great way to defend yourself against a hangover.

For centuries China has praised the benefits of its native plant, and tea drinking has played an integral part in Eastern cultures – not only in China, but also in India and Japan. Today we are discovering what all the fuss was about. Research shows that regular tea drinking promotes healthy bones, skin and teeth, while its vital compounds give protection against serious diseases such as cancer and diabetes. This is particularly true for green tea, which is packed with health-giving flavonoids as well as vitamins and minerals. Its caffeine content is also negligible.

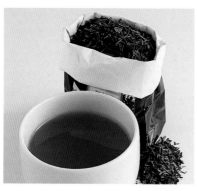

▲ *Green tea is packed with goodness and will help your body return to health.*

powerful properties

Green tea is a potent antioxidant with antibacterial and anti-inflammatory properties. It is also an immunity booster and helps keep you fighting fit so that your body is better able to process harmful substances. It has a cooling, cleansing action on your body and drinking it after you've over-indulged will help your system deal with the toxic overload while soothing any gastric upsets. It also has a head-clearing effect and will help you focus on the day ahead.

There are many varieties of green tea to choose from. Take your pick from Chinese green jasmine, Japanese bancha or sencha, or a green Assam or Darjeeling from India. Look out for and experiment with new green teas as they come onto the market and decide which ones you like best. The secret of a successful green tea brew is to let the water cool off for about five minutes after boiling before pouring it on to the tea and then leaving the tea to steep for about a minute. As a preventative measure, drink two or three cups of green tea a day; for a hangover, drink as much as you can.

122 meadowsweet tisane

A tisane is a type of herbal infusion. This one is made with meadowsweet, a powerful remedy for neutralizing stomach acid. It should help ease many nasty hangover symptoms.

Meadowsweet (*Filipendula ulmaria*) is one of the best antacid remedies for indigestion and heartburn and makes a very useful hangover remedy. It relieves embarrassing and painful wind and flatulence, stems diarrhoea and soothes intestinal spasms. It also has a protective and healing action on the bowel's mucous membranes. Nicholas Culpeper, the 17th-century English herbalist, claimed that meadowsweet was of great help to those that were 'troubled with the cholic, being boiled in wine'.

pain-relieving properties

The herb has a powerful anti-inflammatory and pain-relieving action, which is attributed to the salicylate compounds found in the plant's flowering tops and leaves. When oxidized these compounds yield salicylic acid, from which acetyl-salicylic acid or aspirin can be derived. However unlike aspirin, meadowsweet also contains other constituents that protect the stomach lining while soothing painful, inflamed conditions.

To make a meadowsweet tisane, steep 25g/1oz dried herb or 40g/1½oz fresh herb in 600ml/1 pint/2½ cups of hot water, cover and infuse for about 10 minutes. This is enough to make a pot. For an extra boost, you could also try adding two to three dried clove buds to the pot. Cloves also help to reduce gas and have analgesic properties. They will give the brew a spicy lift.

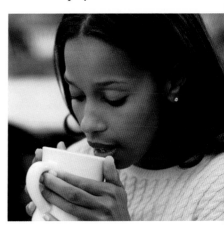

▲ Meadowsweet has analgesic properties. Drink it in a herbal infusion.

123 natural live yogurt

The main reason that your stomach feels as though you are sailing the ocean waves is because its delicate pH balance has been upset. Live yogurt to the rescue.

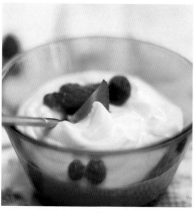

▲ *Eating live yogurt before you go out drinking can help prevent a hangover.*

Overindulgence in alcohol can cause gastritis. This is the official name for an inflammation of the stomach lining and typical symptoms include nausea, vomiting, some abdominal pain, diarrhoea and wind. Excessive alcohol consumption makes your stomach highly acidic – think green bile slopping around – which is why you feel so sick. Yogurt is an alkaline food that will help redress the balance. To work effectively, the yogurt needs to be 'live' and natural and preferably not flavoured or sweetened.

stomach soother

Eating plenty of live yogurt before you go out on a drinking spree may actually help prevent a hangover. It will line your stomach and help protect it from the acidic onslaught later on. Drinking milk has a similar effect, but live yogurt is much better because it contains natural probiotics. These are the 'friendly' bacteria that live in your intestines and are responsible for its healthy workings. It is estimated that your intestines contain about 11 trillion bacteria, 70 per cent of which should be the healthy, probiotic type. Excess alcohol, together with smoking and stress, upsets this balance.

If you didn't manage to eat yogurt before you went out, eating it after you've been drinking is the next best thing. It will soothe and cool your angry insides and help you to feel more human. If you're not keen on the taste of natural yogurt, stir in a little runny honey to sweeten. Remember that honey is also a natural antibiotic and helps the body to metabolize alcohol. It also helps alleviate a thumping headache.

eat your oats

Oats are a top-class 'A' grade food. They are not only rich in nutrients but are also easily digested. Because oats are an alkaline food they are soothing for an upset stomach.

It is estimated that a 90g/3½oz serving of oats contains 15g/½oz of protein. Oats are also rich in calcium, magnesium, iron and potassium and contain plenty of the B-complex vitamins. Being a wholegrain food they are high in fibre that will help to 'bulk' up the contents of your stomach (assuming there are any left) and settle things down. Traditionally oats are used in convalescence to help the body return to health. In days gone by, an oat posset made with oatmeal, water, lemon juice, sugar and spices was a standard prescription in the sickroom.

The soothing and fortifying effect of oats is not only good for your digestive tract but also your nervous system. Oats can help calm jangled nerves and lift your mood so that you feel ready to face the day with poise and grace. Oats cooked as porridge make a great start to the day. To make one serving of porridge, a 40g/1½oz serving of oats should be sufficient, unless you are very hungry.

▶ *Oats can be eaten raw in muesli or cooked and made into porridge.*

hangover muesli mix
To make a supply of homemade muesli you will need:
300g/11oz porridge oat flakes
115g/4oz malted wheat flakes
115g/4oz rye flakes
75g/3oz each of dried apricots, dates, walnuts and almonds
an airtight container

Pour the flakes into the container. Cut up the apricots and dates into small pieces, break up the nuts and add the lot to the oat base and mix well together. The muesli will keep for two to three months. You can experiment by using different fruits and nuts.

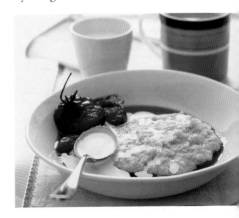

Eat plenty of **fresh fruit** to cleanse and rehydrate your system. **Apples, melons, kiwis** and all the **citrus fruits** are excellent.

126 sprouted seeds

For a powerhouse of goodness there is nothing to beat sprouted seeds. They contain all the plant's nutrients in a highly concentrated form and are fantastic energy boosters.

Excess alcohol really does put an enormous strain on your system. The next day it is almost impossible not to feel tired and irritable from lack of sleep, and suffer the ghastly after-effects as your body struggles to cope with toxic overload. It is no wonder that you feel like death warmed up.

hangover busting sprouts
Sprouted seeds are bursting with life. Eating them will give you energy and help your system to clean out. They are also cheap and easy to grow.

Special sprouters are available in good health stores, or alternatively you can use a large glass jar. To sprout seeds, spread a fine layer over the shelves of a sprouter or put a handful into a jar. Keep them in a light but cool spot, out of direct sunlight and water twice a day. If you are using a jar, cover the top with a mesh 'lid' made from a piece of muslin or nylon stocking. Drain off the water after watering so that the seeds are not left to lie in water. After a day or so, tiny shoots will appear. You can continue to grow the seeds for several days,

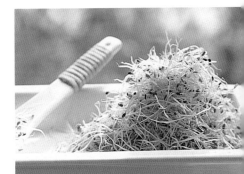

▲ Alfalfa sprouts are easy to grow and have a cleansing action on the body.

harvesting along the way. You can also buy seeds ready sprouted in supermarkets and health stores.

Some of the best seeds to sprout for a hangover are alfalfa or sunflower. Sunflower seeds strengthen your eyes' sensitivity to light and are a potent detoxifier. Alfalfa contains potassium and other minerals and has an anti-inflammatory and cleansing effect on the body. Although not a seed, mung beans are also a good choice. They are rich in minerals, B and C vitamins and are excellent for detoxification. They're also one of the easiest 'seeds' to sprout.

127 hangover breakfasts

If you can face it, a full-protein breakfast – eggs, bacon, sausages, hash browns and the like – is a tried and tested hangover cure that many hangover sufferers swear by.

Think breakfast, think big. Everyone has their favourite version of what they like in a full cooked breakfast, but the number one ingredient has to be an egg or two (or even three).

wholesome eggs

Eggs supply first-class protein, zinc and B vitamins, as well as other nutrients. They are easily digested when lightly boiled, although how people like their eggs cooked varies greatly. Fried eggs are probably the most naughty, but poached eggs will give you a yolk to dip into without the grease factor. Scrambled eggs are another good option.

spicy scrambled egg

2–3 ripe but firm tomatoes
1 small red pepper (capsicum)
1 small yellow pepper
1 green chilli
salt and pepper
Tabasco sauce
6 eggs
120ml / 4fl oz / ½ cup milk
sunflower oil

Skin and chop the tomatoes. Deseed the peppers and the chilli and chop them into small pieces. Beat the eggs with the milk and season with salt and pepper and a dash of Tabasco. Heat the oil in a large frying pan and stir-fry the tomatoes, peppers and chilli briefly. Stir in the egg blend and cook over a low heat until piping hot.

◀ Dishes like spicy scrambled egg are ideal served in a split and toasted baguette.

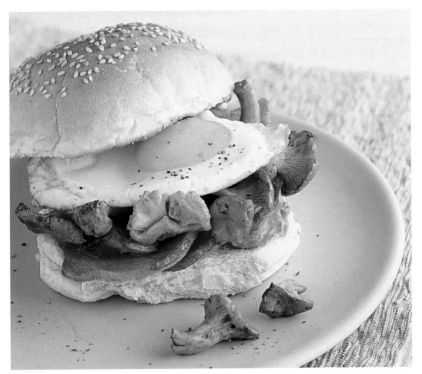

▲ *Bacon, egg and mushroom is a great tasting and nutritious breakfast combination.*

the full monty

Fans of the full-protein breakfast insist that it just 'hits the spot'. If you can keep it inside you after a night on the tiles, it will certainly keep you going for the rest of the day.

In addition to eggs, the other traditional ingredients of the big breakfast include meats such as bacon, sausages and black pudding (blood sausage), although in some parts of the world, beefsteak is popular. Fried potatoes such as hash browns or potato wedges are also on the menu, while fried tomatoes, mushrooms and baked beans add further bulk and flavour. The whole lot is usually accompanied by several slices of fried or toasted bread, and then washed down with a mug of tea or coffee. For those with a sweet tooth, another round of toast topped with marmalade follows this serving of flavoursome comfort fodder.

The easiest way to cook this type of breakfast is to fry the ingredients all together in a single big frying pan. If you are concerned about your figure and/or your cholesterol intake, poach the eggs and cook all the other ingredients under the grill (broiler), although this will mean extra washing up. If you can't face cooking and clearing up, then spoil yourself and head for the nearest café.

128 super soups

Hangover sufferers unable to face up to a square meal may be tempted by a bowl of soup. Soups are quick to prepare, packed with nutrients and help to rehydrate the body.

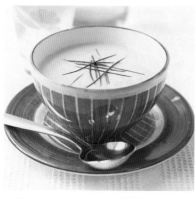

▲ *Freshly made hangover chicken soup is easy on your digestive system.*

Following a heavy night, fragile constitutions will need cosseting and building up. As well being delicious and easy to digest, these wholesome soups are packed with nourishing vitamins and minerals and will boost energy levels.

hangover chicken soup

This hearty, appetizing soup contains barley, which consists of plenty of B-complex vitamins, potassium and other minerals. It also has a soothing action on the stomach, intestines and urinary tract.

1 large onion
15ml/1 tbsp olive oil
1 large carrot
4 sticks celery
1 litre/1¾ pints/4 cups
    chicken stock
1 bay leaf
ground black pepper
25ml/1½ tbsp pot barley
2–3 handfuls bite-sized, cooked
    chicken pieces, without the skin

Chop the onion and soften in the olive oil over a low heat, without letting the onion brown. Wash the rest of the vegetables and chop them into small pieces. Add them to the onion, cover and leave all the vegetables to soften for 5–10 minutes. Check the pan every now and again and give it a stir to make sure the vegetables are not sticking. Pour in the stock and add the bay leaf and enough ground black pepper to taste. Wash the barley and add to the pot, together with the chicken pieces. Bring to the boil, lower the heat and simmer for 1 hour. Check the seasoning and serve with wholemeal bread.

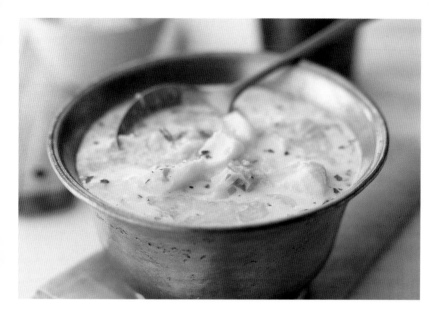

▲ *Soups made with easily digested ingredients will boost energy levels after a hangover.*

Cullen skink soup

This wonderfully comforting soup originates from Cullen, a fishing village in Scotland.

900g/2lb undyed smoked haddock
1 onion, finely sliced
450ml/¾ pint/scant 2 cups milk
450ml/¾ pint/scant 2 cups water
450g/1lb floury potatoes, peeled
    and cut into large chunks
225g/8oz leeks, finely sliced
300ml/½ pint/1¼ cups single
    (light) cream
1 large (US extra large) egg yolk
30ml/2 tbsp chopped fresh parsley
50g/2oz/¼ cup butter
salt and ground black pepper

Put the haddock, skin-side up, in a shallow pan and cover with the onion slices, milk and water. Bring to just below boiling, turn down the heat and poach gently for about 10 minutes until cooked. Meanwhile, boil the potatoes in salted water for 10–15 minutes, or until tender, then drain and mash. When the fish is cooked, strain the cooking liquid into a pan and reserve. Flake the fish and set aside. Whisk the mashed potato into the reserved fish liquid, stir in the leeks, bring to the boil and simmer for 10 minutes until tender. Whisk the cream and egg yolk together and stir into the soup. Reheat gently, without boiling, until slightly thickened. Gently stir in the reserved flaked fish, season to taste, and heat through. Serve piping hot, dotted with knobs (pats) of butter that will melt over the surface.

129 cleansing avocados

The cleansing effects of avocados help to disperse the ghastly after-effects of the demon drink. If you can't face a big meal, a snack or drink will stimulate your overworked system.

Whilst being highly nutritious, avocados have anti-oxidizing properties which make them good for countering toxicity in the body.

a nourishing food

Avocados are almost a complete food as they contain protein and starch as well as fat. Although their fat content is high, it is monounsaturated, which is thought to lower blood cholesterol levels in the body. Avocados also contain valuable amounts of vitamins C and E, as well as iron, potassium and manganese. An extra bonus is that they are said to improve the condition of the skin and hair.

eating avocados

Avocados are usually eaten raw. Once cut, they should be brushed with lemon or lime juice to prevent discoloration. Avocado halves can be dressed with a vinaigrette, or filled with soured cream sprinkled with cayenne pepper, or hummus. Slices or chunks of avocado are delicious in salads. In Mexico, where they grow in abundance, there are countless dishes based on avocados. Guacamole is the best known, but they are also used in a variety of soups and stews.

avocado smoothie

Halve and pit 2–3 avocados. Scoop out the flesh and place in a blender. Add the juice of a lime, plus a crushed clove of garlic, a handful of ice cubes and about 400ml/14fl oz/1⅔ cups vegetable stock. Process until smooth. Pour the mixture into a large jug (pitcher) and stir in 500ml/14fl oz/1⅔ cups milk and a dash of Tabasco sauce. Once the ingredients are fully blended, serve immediately.

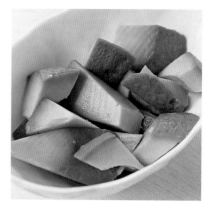

▲ Avocados are good for cleansing the system and help to nourish the skin.

130 homeopathic hanover cures

For a holistic approach to a hangover, choose a homeopathic treatment. Homeopathy considers mental and emotional 'symptoms', as well as the physical ones, and offers suitable remedies.

Homeopathic remedies are prepared from a variety of plants and mineral substances. These are then diluted many times over until no molecules of the original substance remain. It is for this reason that many people are sceptical as to how the remedies can possibly work and put it down to a placebo effect. However homeopathy has been in use for about 200 years, so you will have to decide for yourself whether homeopathy works for you.

homeopathic hangover remedies

The practice of homeopathy is based on the principle that like-cures-like. This means that the symptoms caused by too much of a substance can also be cured by taking a small dose of it. A treatment is selected by matching your symptoms with a suitable remedy. Take the 6C potency, two tablets every hour for six doses. Coffee, peppermint, eucalyptus and other strong smells can antidote homeopathic remedies so are best avoided. Following are some of the best hangover remedies:

• **nux vomica:** the classic hangover remedy. Symptoms brought on by overindulgence in alcohol and rich

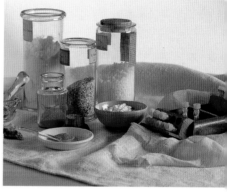

▲ *Homeopathic remedies are taken as small tasteless tablets or as drops.*

food. Sufferer is irritable, impatient, and highly sensitive to light, noises and smells. Absence of thirst.

• **lycopodium:** where there is a lot of gas and heartburn. The sufferer feels better left alone but likes to know there is someone close by.

• **carbo veg:** face pale or sallow; bitter taste in mouth and burning feeling in the stomach; acid indigestion; nausea. Sluggish and irritable; better for fresh air.

• **kali bich:** hangover especially after too much beer; yellow coating on tongue; burning pains in stomach.

131 head massage

A pounding hangover headache can be soothed away with a gentle head massage. It helps to release muscular tension and sends healing signals to the rest of the body.

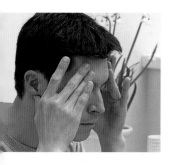

headache soother
1 Use your middle fingers to smooth out your forehead. Use a firm pressure and work from the middle, out towards the hairline. Cover the whole forehead and repeat.

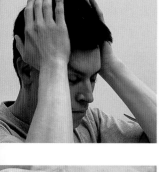

2 Position the heel of your hands over your temples and press inwards with a firm pressure. Using a circling action, work 6 times in a clockwise direction and then repeat 6 times in an anti-clockwise direction.

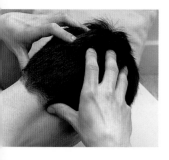

3 Place your thumbs on the bony ridge behind your ears. Use a firm pressure and breathe in. Press and release as you breathe out. Work along the base of the skull until you get to the middle. Repeat 3 times.

Massage is one of the oldest known therapies in the world. Based on the healing power of touch, it can make us feel better almost instantly. Stroking movements appear to trigger the release of endorphins, the body's natural painkillers, and induce feelings of comfort and wellbeing. Studies have also shown that massage is able to strengthen the body's immune system, lower stress levels and speed up the body's elimination of toxins.

massage technique
It is easiest to do the headache massage (left) while sitting at a table so you can support your head with your arms. If you find any particularly tight spots, these are likely to be trigger points for the headache.

quick-fix reflexology

It may not be obvious but you can actually help your hangover by pressing certain reflexology points on your hands or feet, which are like a map in miniature of the whole body.

Pressure applied at certain 'reflex' points on the hands or feet can affect corresponding areas of the body and stimulate natural healing. If energy is flowing freely around your body you will feel well and more positive. In turn your body will respond and its actions will be enhanced. The energy booster (right) will also help strengthen the immune system.

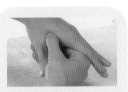

EMERGENCY FIX
There is a special pressure point between the thumb and forefinger that can help to settle an acid stomach and relieve headaches. Use your thumb to press quite hard, exhaling as you do so. Do not do if pregnant.

energy booster
1 To help strengthen the whole body, use your thumb to press firmly around the liver area. This is mid-way along the base of the right foot and is often tender.

2 Now work the digestive area, roughly the middle area of the feet. This area contains pressure points for the liver, stomach, spleen, kidneys and intestines. For sore or tender areas, hold the pressure for a little longer, while breathing out.

3 Finish by working on the upper and lower lymph systems to encourage the speedy removal of toxins. This area is on the top of each foot. Press between the toes with your finger and continue in a line down the foot.

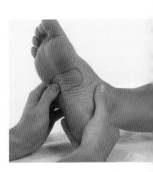

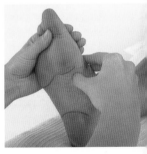

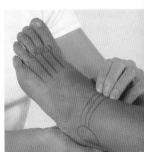

reiki healing

Try a gentle reiki treatment to soothe away your hangover and restore peace and calm. Reiki is a form of hands-on spiritual healing that comes from Japan.

energy therapy

In Japanese, the word 'rei-ki' means universal-life energy. When people give a reiki treatment, they 'channel' this energy. Visualizing it as a white light, they draw it in from the universe through their bodies and allow it to work through their hands.

reiki balancer

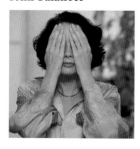

1 Place both hands over closed eyes. Imagine a white light beaming from your hands into your eyes. This should feel refreshing and will clear a heavy head.

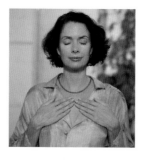

2 Place both hands on your upper chest, visualizing the white light beaming out from them. It may begin to feel warm. This position is good for lymph drainage and for clearing toxins.

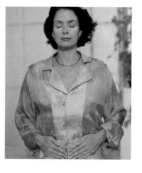

3 Move your hands to your lower abdomen, just below your navel. Continue to visualize the white light as being concentrated beneath your hands. This position transmits healing energy to your stomach and digestive system.

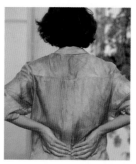

4 Finish with both of your hands resting on your lower back, just over your kidneys. Visualize the white light sending its healing energy to your kidneys and through your body.

crystal magic

It may sound a little far-fetched but crystals and gemstones can be used to exorcize the ill effects of the demon drink. Certain stones have special healing properties.

Crystals are used in healing to work on imbalances in the body's subtle energy system that runs through the body along invisible energy pathways (meridians) and is concentrated at energy hot spots (chakras). When we are ill, the meridians and chakras no longer work properly and our energy becomes stuck or over-stimulated. Feeling good is connected with our vital energies being balanced and flowing freely. This means that a hangover is not only affecting your physical body but is playing havoc with the subtle fine-tuning of your energy body.

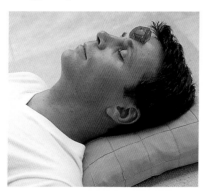

▲ To ease a hangover headache, try an amethyst crystal on your brow chakra.

To treat a hangover headache, place a stone on your brow chakra (the mid-point between the eyebrows); for an upset stomach, on the solar plexus chakra (just above the navel); to help with dehydration, on the lower abdomen chakra (just below the navel); or for low energy and general rebalancing, one on the root chakra (on the pubic bone) and one on the crown chakra (on top of your head).

hangover easing gemstones
There are many different kinds of crystals, each having particular associations and healing properties.
• **clear quartz:** for that groggy 'just let me die' feeling. Quartz strengthens, cleanses and purifies and is a good all-round rebalancer.
• **amethyst:** for a pounding headache and acid indigestion. Amethyst is calming and soothing and is said to be a cure for drunkenness.
• **garnet:** detoxifier, cleanses the blood.
• **citrine:** soothes digestive upsets; also good for liver, kidneys and colon.
• **tourmeline**: has a special affinity with the liver and kidneys; it also cleanses and strengthens.

135 flower essences

There are several flower essences that can help alleviate the symptoms of a hangover. They work primarily on a 'soul' level and help to realign the body's subtle energies when you are sick.

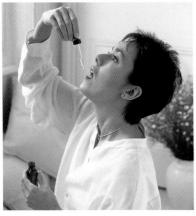

▲ *Flower essence drops can be taken directly from the dropper bottle, or can be added to a glass of water or fresh juice.*

Flower essences are especially useful for dealing with negative mental and emotional states. The Bach flowers are probably the most well-known system, although Australian Bush essences are also popular. Both work on an emotional level, harmonizing negative feelings and belief patterns held in the subconscious mind. Tapping into the "wise, old energy" of the world's first and relatively unpolluted continent, Bush essences are unique and fast acting.

Flower remedies are prepared by infusing flower heads in water, which is believed to absorb the flower's unique vibrations. The liquid is then preserved in brandy.

hangover healers

To treat a hangover, crab apple is probably the number one remedy as it is the essence for cleansing and eliminating toxicity in mind, body and soul. Its purifying effects help to remove negativity. Hornbeam can also be helpful, particularly if you wake with a heavy head and that 'Monday morning feeling'. Hornbeam's energies have been described as a cool, refreshing shower. If you suffer hangovers a little too often, take chestnut bud (4–6 drops 3 times a day) as a preventative – it is the remedy for those who keep repeating the same mistakes.

For acute symptoms, try Bach's rescue remedy or Australian Bush emergency essence. Both contain essences designed to cope with emergency situations. Take 4 drops in a little water every half an hour until your hangover symptoms subside.

The power of colour to influence mood is well known. When you're far from feeling 'in the pink', try some colour therapy to knock your hangover on the head.

Making ourselves feel better with colour is something that we do instinctively. We all know what it's like to have colour fads and how wearing a particular shade can feel just right one day but all wrong the next. Yet our choices may be based on more than a whim as different colours emit different vibrations. Remember that colour is actually light and moves in waves. Darker colours have a longer wavelength and a lower frequency, while lighter colours have a shorter wavelength and higher frequency.

The most obvious way of using colour therapeutically is to wear it as an item of clothing. Another way is to 'bathe' in coloured light by placing a special coloured gel or slide in front of a high-powered lamp, making sure that it is not touching the bulb. You can also make a colour infusion by putting coloured stones or any other colourfast item into a bowl of mineral water and leaving it to infuse for several hours, preferably in sunlight. Pour the water into a glass and drink it. Always make sure that the coloured item you are using is clean before you soak it.

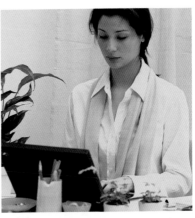

▲ When you're feeling under the weather, surround yourself with healing colours. Green is both detoxifying and refreshing.

colours for a hangover

You can use colour vibrations to treat many hangover symptoms. Hot reds, pinks and oranges are best avoided as they may be over-stimulating.

• **yellow:** digestive disturbances; acid indigestion, sickness, diarrhoea.
• **green:** detoxifying, cleansing.
• **blue, violet:** strengthens and protects the liver; insomnia.
• **turquoise:** immunity booster; anti-inflammatory.
• **indigo:** headaches; painkiller.

The perfect answer! Float away without any effort, your body suspended in warm water in an environment free from external stimuli – no noise, no light. Absolute bliss.

Flotation therapy was developed in the United States during the 1970s. It involves floating in a special sound- and light-proof tank or chamber, although you can switch a light on and open the door at any time. The water is maintained at skin temperature (34.2°C/93.5°F) and contains salts and minerals so that you can float without any effort at all. The result is deep relaxation for both body and mind.

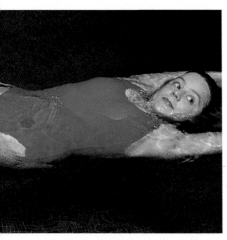

▲ Floating is profoundly relaxing and helps the body to detox. Book yourself a session at your nearest health centre.

mind and body detox

During relaxation, your brain releases endorphins, which are the body's natural painkillers. Many people find flotation to be an uplifting experience similar to meditation. It also helps the body to detox and is a great way of helping to clear a hangover. Floating is probably best tried later on in the day when any acute hangover symptoms, such as sickness and diarrhoea, have subsided. Floating is also a good immunity booster so it should help get you back on your feet in no time.

Most good health clubs have flotation facilities. There is usually a suite of private rooms containing the tank and shower facilities. The tank itself is large enough so that you can comfortably stretch out your arms and legs and the water is usually not very deep – about 30cm (1ft) is sufficient. You can float naked or wear a bathing suit depending on your preference and the club's house rules. After a flotation session, drink plenty of mineral water to help your body flush out and rehydrate. Then take it easy for a few hours to recuperate.

138 aromatherapy massage

Essential oils have powerful healing properties.
Both fennel and juniper are potent detoxifiers
and are wonderful for a hangover. Use them
in an aromatherapy self-massage.

fennel oil

According to folklore, fennel was believed to offer protection against the evil eye. Today the plant's essential oil is recognized for its effectiveness in counteracting the effects of alcoholic poisoning: it has been used successfully in the treatment and rehabilitation of alcoholics. This may be because fennel is a diuretic and a powerful detoxifier. It also has a calming effect on an upset digestive system and gives speedy relief from nausea and acid indigestion.

juniper oil

When the body needs to detoxify, juniper is ideal. It stimulates the body into throwing off toxic wastes and, like fennel, is a diuretic. Juniper is also good for cleansing and purifying on a mental and emotional level, helping to clear away any negativity picked up during social interaction.

Juniper has a strong smell that is surprisingly pleasant when diluted and used in blends. Its characteristic smoky note combines well with the fresh, aniseed-like aroma of fennel. To treat a hangover, one of the best ways of using the oils is through massage.

Essential oils should never be used directly on the skin but mixed in a suitable carrier base, such as sweet almond oil or an unscented lotion. Add 5 drops of fennel and 3 drops of juniper to 30ml/2 tbsp oil or lotion and mix well. If you wish, you could also add a couple of drops of lemon oil to give it a refreshing, citrus tang. Massage the oil into your thighs, upper back, arms and shoulders using smooth, circling movements.

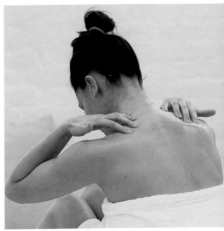

▲ Use essential oils of juniper, fennel and lemon in an aromatherapy massage. It will help with your hangover detox.

139 aching head easer

Two of the best essential oils for a hangover headache are lavender and peppermint. When used together they make a formidable combination. You can use them in a balm.

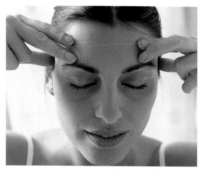

▲ *Gently rub a little balm into your temples with your fingertips for headache relief.*

The most important constituent of peppermint oil is menthol. When your head is heavy and you can't think straight, the smell of peppermint is like a breath of fresh air that will blow away the cobwebs. Lavender oil also has a refreshing aroma, although its effect is more calming and balancing.

Both peppermint and lavender oils are anti-inflammatory with analgesic (pain-relieving) properties. They are complementary to one another, each enhancing the action of the other. Peppermint is a stimulant and lavender a sedative. This combination of stimulant and sedative is found in many commercial pain-killing preparations but there is an important difference: essential oils not only kill the pain but they also get to work on its underlying causes. Used correctly, they are also non-toxic.

lavender and peppermint balm
To ease a hangover headache, make up your own lavender and peppermint balm and keep it on standby. Use 3 drops each of lavender and peppermint to every 60ml/4 tbsp unscented base cream. Blend the oils into the cream and keep in a screw-top jar. When you need to use, massage a little into your temples.

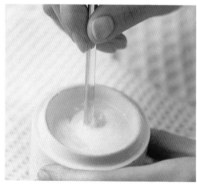

▲ *It is easy to make up a headache balm using lavender and peppermint oils.*

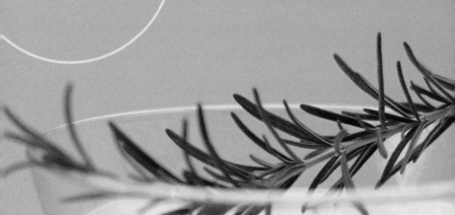

Wake up your senses with the clean, sharp smell of rosemary. Vaporize a few drops of the essential oil in a burner for an instant hangover cure to leave you refreshed and ready for a new day.

141 revitalizing bath oil

Grapefuit is undeniably refreshing whilst coriander is soothing. Their amazing properties will soon restore you – particularly when combined with a relaxing warm bath.

After a night partying, a refreshing, restorative bath containing grapefruit and coriander oils will soon have you back on your feet.

Extracted from the fruit's fresh peel, grapefruit oil has cleansing, balancing, brightening and refreshing properties that ease muscle fatigue and stiffness as well as soothe headaches and nervous exhaustion. It can also have a beneficial effect on a digestion that has been upset by over-indulgence in alcohol, as it helps to

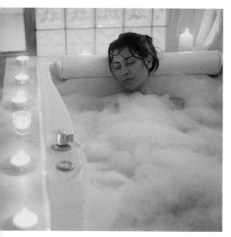

▲ *Bathing in a grapefruit and coriander bath should help restore your equilibrium.*

break down fatty foods and cleanses the kidneys. A good all-rounder, this uplifting oil is also used to treat colds, flu, chills, apathy and PMS.

The essential oil of coriander has calming, soothing properties and it is also thought to be useful for the repair skin tissues.

grapefruit and coriander bath oil
This stimulating and refreshing combination of oils is a great reviver and will help you recover from the debilitating effects of a hangover. Add one tablespoon to the bath water immediately before you step into it, otherwise the oils will evaporate before they have had a chance to adhere to your skin.

100ml/3½fl oz almond oil
20ml/4tsp wheatgerm oil
30 drops grapefruit essential oil
30 drops coriander essential oil

Pour the almond oil and wheatgerm oil into a 120ml/4fl oz opaque glass bottle. Add the essential oils and gently shake to mix. Store in the dark and use within six months.

142 citrus spritzer

When you want the world to stop, a fragrant mist of citrus scents will refresh your spirits and give you a boost. It's an instant quick fix that is easy to prepare.

When life has to go on regardless of how you feel, an emergency quick-fix solution is called for.

Without having to eat or drink a single thing, a quick burst of on-the-spot aromatherapy can give you a lift and change your mood. Whether or not you are aware of it, different scents influence the way that you feel. This is because your sense of smell is registered in the area of the brain that is associated with moods, emotions and instinctive responses. Citrus scents are refreshing, tangy and revitalizing. A handy way of using them is in a mist-sprayer.

emergency reviver

For an instant energizer, make a mix containing three distinctive, but complementary, citrus scents: lemon, grapefruit, and bergamot. Bergamot oil is one of the essential ingredients in eau-de-Cologne toilet water and is what gives Earl Grey tea its distinctive scent and flavour. It is uplifting and reviving. The fresh, clean, lively scent of lemon dispels sluggishness and will put you in a better frame of mind, while the tangy,

sweet aroma of grapefruit will also lighten your mood and give you a kick start into action. To make a mist-spray add 150ml/¼ pint/⅔ cup water to a spray bottle (tap water is fine). Then add 6 drops of bergamot and 5 drops each of lemon and grapefruit. Shake the bottle well before you spray to help the oil droplets disperse. Hold the mister about 30cm/1ft away from you and spritz away. Make sure that you do not spray directly on to your eyes or any polished surfaces.

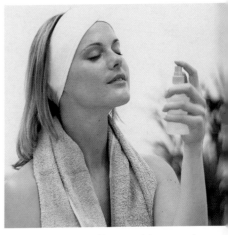

▲ An aromatic mist of bergamot, lemon and grapefruit is an instant pick-me-up.

143

chamomile compress

When you have a hangover you need to be especially gentle with yourself. Chamomile is one of the mildest and most soothing of all the essential oils. Give it a try.

In Ancient Egypt, the chamomile plant was dedicated to the sun god, Ra, for its effectiveness in bringing down a fever. Chamomile is soothing and anti-inflammatory, which makes it especially useful for dealing with excess heat in the body. Too much alcohol aggravates the body's delicate internal balance and produces an acid, over-heated system. This not only shows up on a physical level but also affects mood and emotions. With a hangover, acid indigestion and

sickness is often accompanied by irritability and anxiety and these are all signs that the body is under stress.

Chamomile is one of the best remedies for a generally upset system. It is especially effective for digestive disorders, particularly when stomach cramps and diarrhoea are present. On a mental level, it is calming and soothing for all states of anger or agitation. Like lavender, chamomile's overall effect is to rebalance the body's energies and restore harmony.

stomach soothing compress
If your hangover is accompanied by griping stomach pains and you feel generally unwell, a chamomile compress over your abdomen is a gentle but effective treatment. To make the compress you need a piece of clean cotton cloth and a bowl of hand-hot water. About 300ml/ ½ pint/1¼ cups water should be sufficient. Add 6 drops of chamomile to the water and stir well. Soak the cloth in the water, allowing it to absorb the oils. Squeeze it lightly and position it over your abdomen for 10–15 minutes. Lie back and relax.

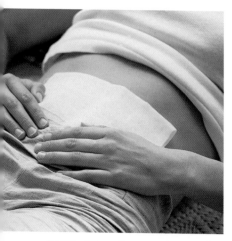
▲ *A warm chamomile compress over your abdomen can relieve stomach pains.*

144 aromatic facial

Frequent excessive drinking is ageing and damaging to your complexion. Give your face a morning-after treat with an aromatic facial – a steam followed by a rich moisturizer.

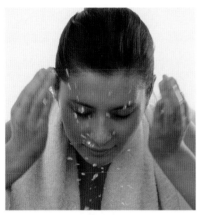

▲ *Splashing your face with water will leave your skin tingly and refreshed.*

You may not be aware of it, but your face will eventually register the telltale signs of all your alcoholic binges. Drinking a lot of alcohol puts pressure on the delicate blood vessels in your face. Constant dilation of these vessels strains the fibrous connective tissue and the vessel walls will eventually collapse, with your skin losing its suppleness and elasticity. Dehydration caused by drinking will also take its toll: your skin will dry out and any facial lines will look more pronounced.

refreshing facial

If this doesn't sound too good, then it's a good idea to minimize the damage by giving your skin an extra nourishing treat after you've been out on the town. An aromatic facial uses essential oils in various ways. A good place to start is with a steam treatment. Put 2–3 drops of geranium oil in a bowl of near-boiling water. Close your eyes and sit in the steam for about five minutes. For a stronger effect, you could also make a 'tent' with a towel draped over your head and the bowl to capture the steam. The steam will open your pores while geranium is cleansing and refreshing for all skin types.

Once your skin feels clean, splash your face with some icy cold spring water to close the pores. By now your skin should feel tingly and be beginning to lose its death-mask appearance. Leave your skin to settle for 15 minutes or so before applying a rich moisturizer. For a nourishing and rejuvenating cream, mix 4 drops of rose and 2 drops of frankincense with 60ml/4 tbsp unscented base cream. Store in a screw-top jar.

Hangovers are heavy on the eyes.

Try the classic

cucumber cure

– lie back with a slice of cucumber

over each eye and that nasty

puffy red look should just disappear.

Cucumbers are cooling and

refreshing and contain

valuable properties that help the eyes.

146 take it easy

Having a hangover is nature's way of saying 'stop'. Your body needs a chance to rest and recuperate and you have every excuse to stay at home and take it easy.

Admit it, there's a part of you that's secretly glad that you feel so bad. It means no work, no one to tell you what to do, and an excuse to lie back with your feet up. So take the phone off the hook, listen to some relaxing music, graze on snacks and watch television or a video. If you feel up to it, you may even want to read – but nothing too strenuous, perhaps your favourite magazine or that paperback that's been lying around for ages.

rest your over-worked system

Before you start to feel guilty, remember that a hangover puts an enormous strain on your body. You are severely dehydrated and your brain seems to have shrunk to the size of a walnut. Without moving a muscle, your liver and kidneys are working overtime to pump out the poisons, your heart is working extra hard and you are losing valuable nutrients. On top of it all, you didn't sleep well last night. You tried drinking black coffee to sober you up but all that did was keep you awake. When you lay down you felt giddy and had to get up and run to the bathroom. This morning you had to clean it up. It's no wonder you feel so gruesome.

So stop fighting and give in. Keep your fluid intake high, eat something nutritious (if you can) and let nature take its course. The effects of a hangover last about 24 hours so be patient – you'll soon feel better and ready to do it all over again.

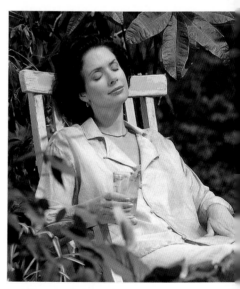

▲ A hangover is the perfect excuse to sit back, relax and put your feet up.

147 pump it out

If you work out regularly you'll find that your hangover recovery time is shortened. Once you're over the very worst of it, you may even feel like taking some exercise.

feel the benefit

Everyone knows that exercise is good for you. It boosts circulation, increases [heart] rate and builds stamina and s[trong] muscles. It is also one of the be[st way]s of releasing stress. When you are [stre]ssed, the body produces extr[a adr]enaline as its fight/flight mec[hanism] gets triggered. When this is not [used] up, it gets stored in your body a[s a] waste. Vigorous exercise (the kind that makes you sweat) helps your body to release toxins, leading to a natural 'high', because it raises your endorphin levels, lifting your spirits and making you feel better. It also builds immunity and helps you recover faster when you do get sick.

know your limitations

Exercising will help you recover from a hangover but only if you work within your 'feel-good' limits. Now is not the time to start working-out with a vengeance if you are not used to it. Take a walk in the fresh air or dig the garden for an hour or so. You could also try cleaning and tidying up the house as that will get your circulation moving without being too taxing. Once you are on the road to recovery, you may feel up to doing something a little more vigorous. Choose an activity that you enjoy, such as going to the gym, power walking, jogging, dancing, cycling or swimming. It will help your body get rid of any lingering toxins and really knock your hangover on its head. Remember to drink plenty of water.

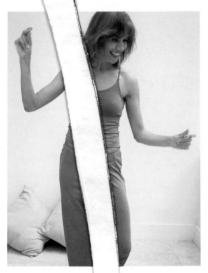

▲ *Dancing is fun. It keeps you fit and helps you to get over a hangover faster.*

148 mind-bending meditation

One of the good things about meditation is that it can give you a natural lift without any nasty repercussions later. It is also healing for mind, body and soul.

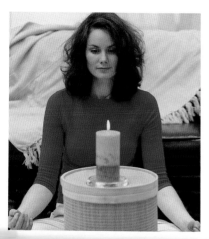
Meditation helps bring you back into

The good news is that even ten minutes of meditation can work wonders and minimize the damage. The following meditation uses sound.

humming meditation

Certain sounds send relaxing signals to body and mind. This meditation uses humming which sets up a healing vibration in your body. Sit in a quiet spot where you won't be disturbed and make yourself comfortable. Your spine needs to be as straight as possible, but make sure your back is well supported. Close your eyes and

you tend to feel like death warmed up – and that's without the drinking. Add alcohol to the mix and it's no wonder you feel so grim.

humming stops, sit quietly for another five minutes continuing to visualize the golden light filling your body. Get up slowly at the end.

149 get intimate

When you and your partner both have the hangover from hell, what better way to commiserate than by getting intimate with one another. It could make you both feel better.

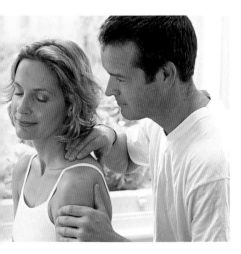

◀ *Touch is one of the best natural therapies of all. Try it with your partner.*

sensual healing

Being stroked, rubbed or touched in a sensitive, loving way not only feels good, but also triggers the release of endorphins, your body's natural analgesics or painkillers. It also boosts circulation and helps to oxygenate your blood, improving the flow of vital nutrients through your body. Massage improves lymphatic drainage and stimulates the removal of toxins. It also boosts immunity, eases muscular tension and dissolves energy blocks so that your body's natural healing energies can freely flow.

Although sex is probably the last thing on your mind right now, you could start off with a little touch therapy. Touch is an instinctive response to pain and in the right hands is very healing. Hippocrates, the famous physician from Ancient Greece, recommended that every doctor should be experienced in 'rubbing'. This is because the skin is the body's largest sensory organ. Skin contains thousands of receptors that react to external stimuli by transmitting messages through the nervous system to the brain.

You don't need to know any special strokes to give your partner a massage, but let your intuition be your guide. Who knows – there's every chance that as you relax and start feeling good together, your sexual desire may start to ignite. So give it a try – for sex is one of the best natural therapies of all. Best of all, you can do it without having to get up – and afterwards you may drift into a peaceful slumber.

150

snooze & sleep

Too much booze affects your sleep. The chances are you didn't get very much last night and have woken up feeling like something that the cat dragged in.

To cure a hangover, take a tip from domestic cats. They spend most of their lives asleep. Anytime, anywhere (so long as it's warm) they snooze their way to dreamland, pictures of utter bliss and relaxation.

disturbed sleep

If only it were that simple. You've spent the whole night tossing and turning, up and down to the bathroom. When you fell asleep, the alcohol in your system drugged your brain and interfered with your body's normal sleep pattern. Critically, you were unable to enter the important REM (rapid eye movement) stage that is associated with dreaming and which is critical to a good night's rest. This lack of refreshing dream sleep is one of the reasons why you feel so irritable, bad-tempered and exhausted, along with just about everything else bad that you can think of.

restorative catnaps

Sleep is one of nature's greatest healers. During sleep your body's cells renew and repair themselves and your brain is able to process information.

Sleep is relaxing and rejuvenating and is really one of the best hangover cures of all. So take plenty of catnaps during the day and have an early night. You'll wake up full of bounce and ready to face the world. If you have trouble dropping off, a warm milky drink flavoured with nutmeg can help.

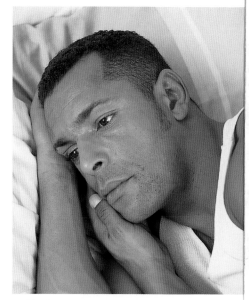

▲ *Give in to tiredness and take a nap. Sleep is probably the simplest, and yet greatest, healer of them all.*

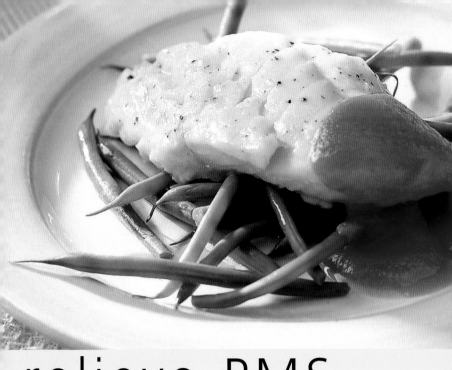

relieve PMS

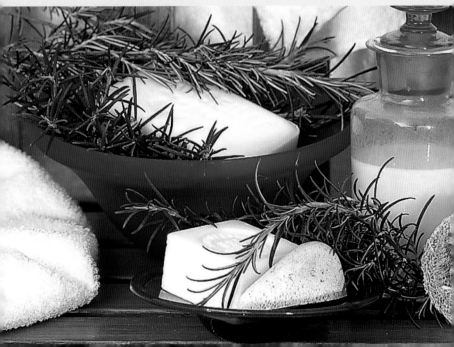

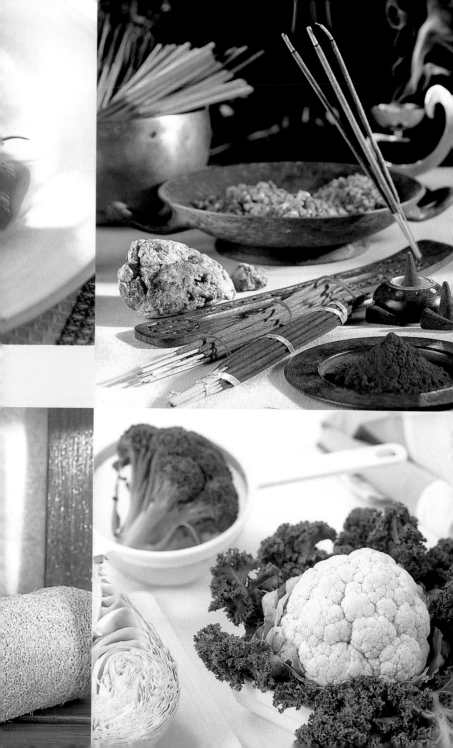

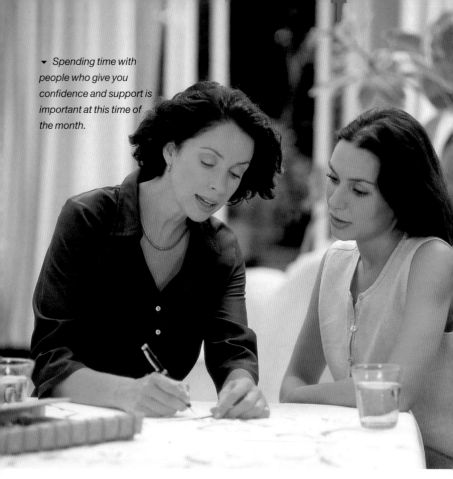

▼ Spending time with people who give you confidence and support is important at this time of the month.

how to ease PMS

Many women dread two weeks out of every month, from the time of ovulation right through to the start of menstruation. Most experience, to some degree, at least some of the large number of symptoms that make up premenstrual syndrome (PMS), from mild discomfort and food cravings, to painful abdominal cramps, headaches and migraine, water retention, nasal congestion or aching limbs.

nutritional aids

Fortunately, there are many ways to alleviate, if not eradicate, PMS conditions. Taking steps to control your diet alone can yield vast improvements. Making sure that you eat a small portion of starchy food every few hours, and taking care to avoid caffeine, alcohol, high-fat and high-sugar foods, will keep your blood sugar on an even keel. This will act to control mood swings and prevent migraines, for example. Fruit juices and smoothies will help curb a tendency to binge on sweet foods, while yogurt containing "friendly" bacteria will help balance the bacteria in your stomach, making for fewer episodes of indigestion and bloating.

Including all the essential vitamins and minerals in your diet – from cramp-relieving vitamin B6 to magnesium, which reduces sugar and chocolate cravings – will go a long way to keeping you feeling your best.

Over the long term, taking supplements such as evening primrose oil and borage oil, which contain essential fatty acids (EFAs), can help balance your hormonal levels and control a wide range of symptoms. Herbal supplements such as feverfew for headaches and peppermint for stomach upsets provide immediate relief.

healthful exercise

Exercise is, of course, important at any time of the month, but it is crucial to stretch the muscles when you are experiencing PMS achiness and tenderness in the tissues. You can reduce high-impact exercises at times when you are feeling tender, and concentrate on gentle stretches, such as Pilates and yoga. Add some simple exercises designed specifically to alleviate discomfort in areas such as the abdomen and back. The legs are another area where it is common to experience premenstrual discomfort; stretching the muscles will ease pain, especially when you are sitting at a desk or at bedtime.

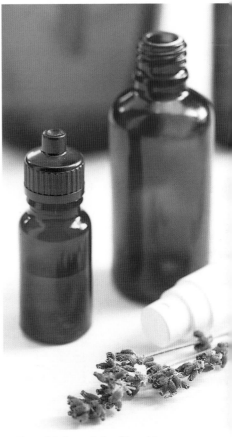

▲ Essential oils can help with a wide range of symptoms, both physical and mental.

soothing treatments

Treatments that use aromatherapy can go a long way towards relieving symptoms. Essential oils such as pine, crampbark and rosemary can soothe painful tissues, while oils such as clary sage and naiouli have been known to help balance female hormones. Incense mixtures can help you achieve a state of calm when your nerves are frayed and you are feeling irritable, and gentle inhalations can ease the sinus congestion and asthma that many women experience during the days preceding menstruation. A dose of pure pleasure, flower oils such as rose and jasmine can help raise the spirits with their delicious and enlivening scents.

palliative measures

There are many therapies that will not only soothe physical discomfort, but also act as system "rechargers". Reflexology is good for relieving built-up pressure in the ovaries, and an abdomen massage will ease cramps, working from the outside in. By practising deep breathing, you will be oxygenating all the cells in your body, thus improving the function of its systems. Solutions such

as homeopathy and crystal healing can balance both physical and emotional systems, while reiki works by directing a positive flow of fast-acting, healing energy from one person to another – and you can also train to use it on yourself.

uplifting attitudes

By keeping a simple chart of your symptoms each month, you can get some idea of the impact PMS has on your life. This will help remind you of why you may not feel your best, and encourage you to be easy on yourself. It will also help you plan important activities for the more high-energy days of the month.

Daily positive affirmations can help boost your confidence levels, while taking measures to enjoy sex fully at a time when your libido level is high can enhance your relationship with your partner. In the modern world, we tend to forget our physical links with nature, but understanding the effect the lunar cycle has on women can be a real eye-opener.

If you get over-emotional, then meditation can help you maintain calm and perspective, as can sound, peaceful sleep at night. The more vivid dreams that accompany this time of heightened awareness can help broaden your experience of self, helping you to accept and enjoy this time as an important aspect of life.

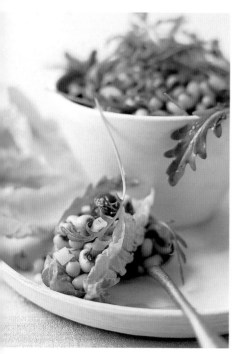

◂ *Legumes such as beans provide the slow-burning carbohydrates and high fibre that help to keep your body's blood sugar levels on an even keel.*

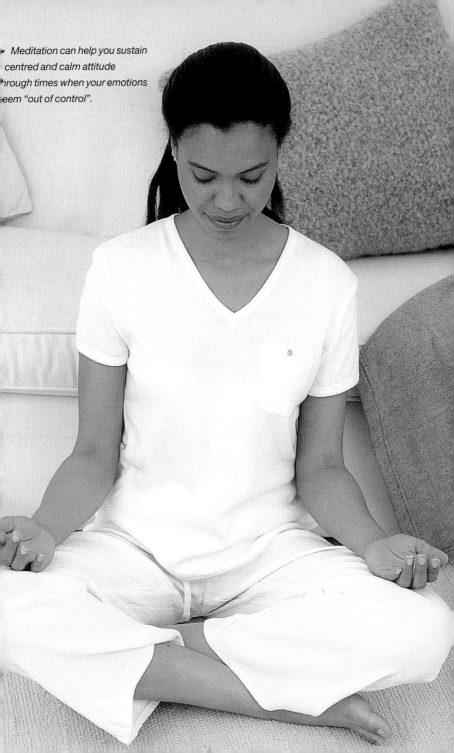

Meditation can help you sustain centred and calm attitude through times when your emotions seem "out of control".

symptom-easing strategies

It is possible to reduce the intensity of premenstrual symptoms by changing the way you eat and drink in the week or so before your period. This section gives you strategies for eating little and often, curbing cravings for sugar and fat, and including nutrients in your diet to ease the discomfort of headaches and migraine, water retention, bloating and tenderness.

Also included are ideas for sensible exercise – from calming yoga to gentle stretches – together with natural therapies that will dispel aches and discomfort in areas such as the back and abdomen. Aromatherapy and herbal treatments not only do wonders for physical symptoms, their fresh scents give you an emotional lift as well.

Because this can be a sensitive time of the month, strategies for dealing with mood swings and handling relationships ensure that minor irritations are dealt with before they become major problems. Finally, tips on boosting your self-esteem and exploring creative activities can help you use this time to your best advantage.

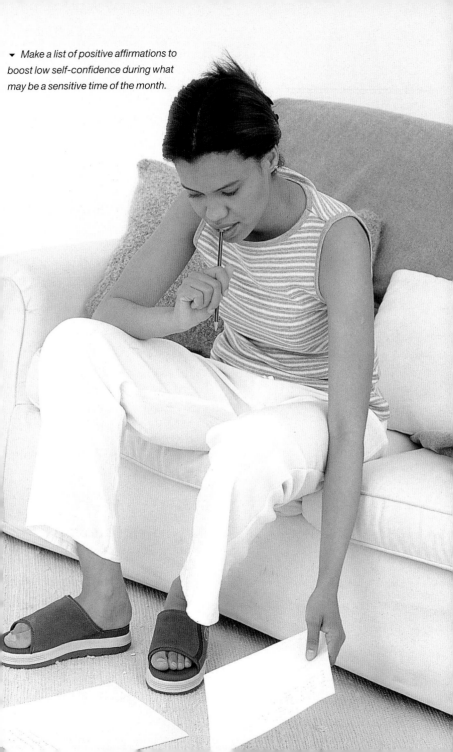

▼ *Make a list of positive affirmations to boost low self-confidence during what may be a sensitive time of the month.*

151 frequent starch diet

Specialists have discovered that following a diet that includes eating starchy food every few hours is the most important thing you can do to keep premenstrual symptoms at bay.

healthy balance

The single most effective and natural way you can help to prevent PMS symptoms is by eating a small amount of starchy food every 3 hours. This will ensure a healthy blood sugar balance, which will in turn ensure that progesterone – an important hormone released by the ovaries and adrenals – is absorbed into the cells. Correct progesterone absorption cannot take place in the cells if adrenaline – the "fight or flight" hormone – is present. If you miss a meal and your blood sugar level dips,

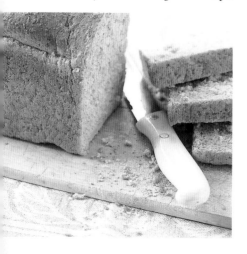

the body suffers from an excess of adrenaline, leading not only to physical symptoms such as water retention and breast tenderness, but also to feelings of irritability, anxiety and confusion.

the diet

Continue to eat well-balanced and nutritious foods, and follow these guidelines during the week before and during a period. Starches to eat include oats, breads, rice, corn, potatoes and rye. They should preferably be whole foods without additives. When you are going out, take snacks with you: if your blood sugar level dips, it takes the body several days to "reclaim" the benefits.
• Morning: eat a starchy food within an hour of waking.
• Daytime: eat a small, starchy snack every 3 hours.
• Evening: eat a starchy food not more than an hour before going to sleep.
• Do not go for more than 10 hours overnight without eating.

◀ *Keep a fresh loaf of bread on hand so that you can quickly prepare starchy snacks.*

152 binge-curbing foods

It is counterproductive to go on an eating spree at any time, but especially just before your period, when blood sugar levels are best kept on an even keel. Some foods can help to prevent bingeing.

Research has shown that you can help to alleviate premenstrual symptoms by decreasing your intake of refined sugar, chocolate, salt and saturated fats. This may be a time when you find that you crave these types of food the most, but you can curb your appetite for them by having healthier foods on hand and eating regularly throughout the day.

snack bowl
Keep a large bowl handy filled with a selection of fresh fruits – for example, bananas, grapes, apples and pears. Their fructose (fruit sugar) content will curb your appetite for the refined sugars in cakes and cookies. Nuts and seeds are also good to keep at hand: they are extremely nutritious and provide healthy plant oils rather than harmful saturated fats.

All vegetables are storehouses of vitamins and minerals. Chop up some crudités – carrots, celery, green and red peppers, spring onions – and put them in a bowl of iced water so that they stay fresh and appetizing. Their crunchy texture will satisfy the need to chew, and keep you from grabbing salty, high-fat snacks.

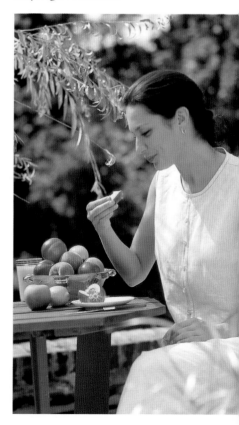

▶ *Fresh fruit is nutritious and will curb your desire for refined sugars.*

153

digestion-aiding yogurt

Stomach upsets can plague PMS sufferers. A simple way to ensure smooth digestion is to include live yogurt in your diet, especially in the week before and during your period.

If you are not in the habit of eating plain yogurt, you'll be surprised at the number of different ways you can incorporate it into your diet. Apart from the traditional muesli and yogurt for breakfast, you can add fresh fruit

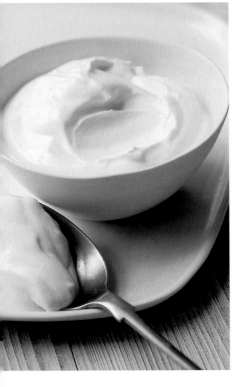

and nuts to plain yogurt, blend it with fruit to make thick smoothies, and mix it with fruit juices to make health-giving drinks.

Yogurt also makes a delicious addition to many savoury dishes. Use it as a garnish to soups, or mix it with chives for a low-fat topping on baked potatoes. Add a dash of mustard to yogurt and use it as a dip for crudités or corn chips. Yogurt makes the perfect base for creamy salad dressings to use on green or potato salads.

home-made yogurt

Bring 600ml/1 pint/2½ cups milk (any kind) to the boil in a pan, remove from the heat and leave to cool to 45°C/113°F, or when the milk feels slightly hotter than is comfortable for a dipped finger. Whisk in 15–30ml/ 1–2 tbsp live yogurt to act as a starter. Transfer to a sterilized bowl and cover with clear film. Insulate the bowl with several layers of dish towels and place in a warm airing cupboard. Leave for 10–12 hours until set.

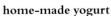

◂ *You can add fruit to plain yogurt or use it in a variety of savoury dips and dressings.*

154 natural sugar sources

Indulging in sugary snacks can send blood sugar levels into orbit during PMS. These healthy juices contain minerals and fructose, burned slowly by the body, to help reduce cravings.

apple and leaf lift-off
This fragrant blend of apple, grapes, fresh green leaves and lime juice is a refreshing rejuvenator.

1 apple
150g/5oz white grapes
small handful of fresh coriander (cilantro), with stalks
25g/1oz watercress or rocket (arugula)
15ml/1 tbsp lime juice

Cut the apple into quarters. Using an extractor, juice the apple, grapes, coriander and watercress or rocket. Add the lime juice to the fruit and herb mixture and stir. Pour into a glass and drink immediately.

fennel fusion
This aromatic combination is full of minerals and vitamins.

½ small red cabbage
½ fennel bulb
2 apples
15ml/1 tbsp lemon juice

▶ *These juices help to reduce cravings and are a healthy alternative to sweet snacks.*

Slice the red cabbage and the fennel into chunks and cut the apple into quarters. Using an extractor, juice the vegetables and fruit. Stir the lemon juice into the mixture and drink immediately.

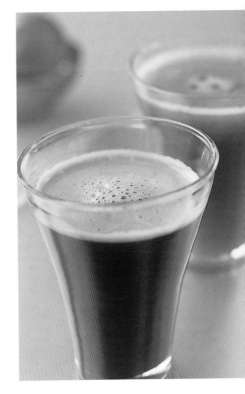

155 cystitis easers

Before and during your period, your urinary tract can be prone to infection. Including cranberry and blueberry in your diet can help prevent cystitis, a bacterial infection of the bladder and urethra.

Cystitis is marked by a burning sensation when urinating, as well as the frequent urge to urinate. It is caused when *E. coli* bacteria bind themselves to the urinary tract lining, and there is an increased tendency for this to occur after sex and during premenstrual and menstruation days. Studies have shown that cranberries can actually inhibit this process, and doctors have long recommended that women include cranberry juice in their diet, both to alleviate and to prevent the condition.

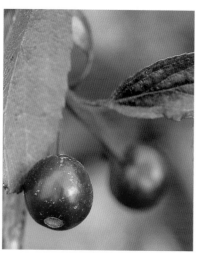

cranberry-blueberry crush
Refreshing cranberries are tart, so you would not want to eat them "straight". Ready-made juices are the easiest option, and are sometimes mixed with apple and raspberry juice. A traditional way to eat the fruit is in cranberry sauce, which is served with turkey, chicken or vegetarian nut roasts.

Blueberries are a powerful anti-oxidant, and also help to reduce the risk of infection. Milder-tasting than cranberries, they can be added straight to yogurt, muesli and cereals. Whizz a handful of blueberries in a blender with cranberry juice and ice for a great, bacteria-busting drink.

supplement options
Because cranberries contain very little sugar, a substantial amount is added to commercial juices. Low-sugar varieties are now available, and cranberry supplements, available from health food stores, are a good way to avoid the extra sugar completely.

◄ *Cranberry juice helps to prevent and ease painful cystitis. It is best to buy ready-made juices because fresh cranberries are tart.*

156

helpful herbal teas

Some herbs act to ease and dispel a variety of PMS symptoms. Instead of coffee or tea – which contain caffeine, known to increase anxiety and discomfort – try these soothing combinations.

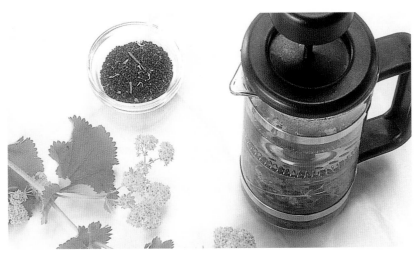

▲ Herbal teas are a gentle way to relieve PMS symptoms, relax the system and lift the mood.

lady's mantle and vervain tea

This herbal infusion is said to be effective in the prevention of heavy bleeding during periods.

Put 5ml/1 tsp each of dried lady's mantle and vervain in a pot, then add 300ml/½ pint/1¼ cups boiling water. Steep for 10 minutes, strain and sweeten to taste with honey or brown sugar. Drink one cup twice a day from day 14 of your monthly cycle (two weeks after the beginning of your period).

rose petal and valerian tea

Good for easing premenstrual insomnia, valerian is a potent relaxer. Rose petals ease pain, lift the spirits and smell lovely.

Place 5ml/1 tsp rose petals in a pot with 2.5ml/½ tsp valerian (you can use the powdered contents of a capsule). Add 300ml/½ pint/1¼ cups boiling water and steep for 5–10 minutes. Add a small amount of honey, or drink unsweetened.

Pluck a
sprig of chamomile
fresh from the garden,
add a slice of lemon, pour on
hot water and drink to
calm the nerves and
quell PMS anger.

158 low-fat comfort food

During the premenstrual countdown, the urge to "pig out" on high-fat foods such as crisps and fries may be immense. This recipe provides the comfort of fries without the harmful fat content.

roasted oven fries

2 large baking potatoes
25ml/1½ tbsp olive oil
5ml/1 tsp fresh herbs such as rosemary and thyme, chopped
scant sprinkling of sea salt (or lemon juice if you are avoiding salt)
low-fat mayonnaise, for dipping

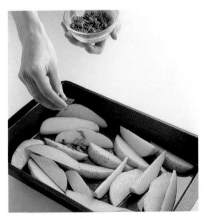

1 Place a roasting pan in the oven and preheat to 240°C/475°F/ Gas 9. Cut the potatoes in half lengthwise, then into thin wedges. When the pan is hot, remove it and put in the oil, potatoes, herbs and sea salt or lemon juice. Toss well to coat the potatoes evenly, spreading them out in a single layer.

2 Roast the potatoes in the oven for 20–25 minutes, turning at least once, until the wedges are golden brown and puffy. Sprinkle with more herbs, if you like, and a little more sea salt or lemon juice to taste. Serve the fries immediately, while hot and crunchy, with low-fat mayonnaise for dipping.

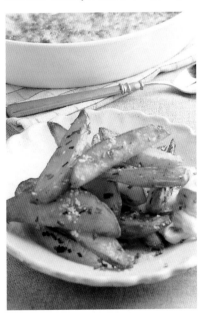

▲ *The hearty crunch and herby taste of these fries satisfies the taste buds.*

159 nutritious vegetables

Poor nutrition is a contributory factor to PMS, which is due to monthly lowered hormone levels in the body. Including plenty of fresh vegetables in your diet will help to keep PMS at bay.

Green leafy vegetables – spinach, spring greens, Brussels sprouts, chard and kale – are packed with nutrients. They contain large amounts of vitamin C, B vitamins, iron (a mineral often depleted monthly in women), zinc and potassium, as well as lots of fibre and cancer-fighting antioxidants. Spinach contains oxalic acid, which inhibits the body's absorption of iron, but eating it together with a vitamin C-rich food will increase absorption. Eat spinach raw in a salad or lightly steamed.

Leafy vegetables are best eaten as soon as possible as they do not keep well – 2 to 3 days at most. Store in a cool, dark area.

▼ *Leafy vegetables are best eaten raw or lightly cooked to retain their flavour and nutrients.*

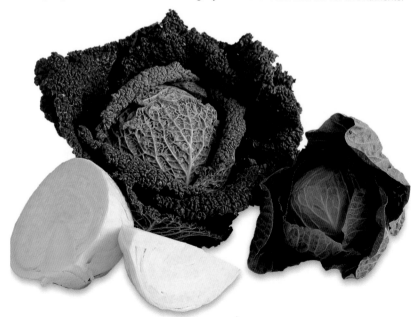

spinach with rice and dill

Serves 4

675g/1½lb fresh spinach
60ml/4 tbsp extra virgin olive oil
1 large onion, chopped
juice of ½ lemon
150ml/¼ pint/⅔ cup water
115g/4oz long grain rice
45ml/3 tbsp chopped fresh dill, plus
   extra sprigs to garnish
ground black pepper
salt

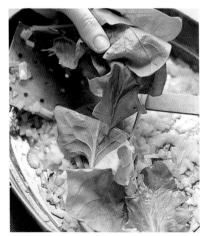

1 Wash the spinach well and drain in a colander. Shake off excess water and shred the leaves coarsely.

2 Heat the olive oil in a large pan and sauté the chopped onion until it is translucent. Add the spinach leaves to the pan and stir for a few minutes to coat with the oil.

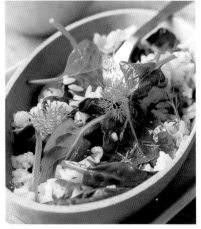

3 As soon as the spinach looks wilted, add the lemon juice and water, and bring to the boil. Add the rice and dill, cover and cook gently for about 10 minutes. If it looks too dry, add a little water. Season to taste.

4 Serve hot or at room temperature, placing sprigs of dill over the top.

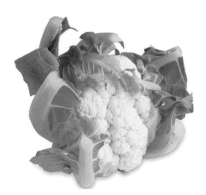

◀ *Eat leafy vegetables as fresh as possible, as tired vegetables will have lost many of their valuable nutrients and flavour. Look for brightly coloured leaves without any signs of yellowing or wilting. Cauliflowers should have a tight, creamy head.*

160 protein-rich fish

Fish such as tuna can contribute essential protein to your PMS diet regime. Low in saturated fat, it is easy to digest and is a good substitute for red meat, which is best avoided before a period.

seared tuna, bean and noodle Niçoise

Serves 4

2 fresh tuna steaks
175g/6oz fine green beans, trimmed
350g/12oz medium dried egg noodles
225g/8oz halved baby plum tomatoes
3 hard-boiled eggs, quartered
50g/2oz black olives
fresh basil leaves, torn

For the dressing:
90ml/6 tbsp olive oil
30ml/2 tbsp lemon juice
2.5ml/½ tsp Dijon mustard
45ml/3 tbsp chopped parsley

Rinse the tuna steaks. Combine the dressing ingredients in a jar, shake to mix and set aside. Blanch the green beans in boiling water for 4 minutes. Drain, place in a bowl with the noodles, and pour boiling water over to cover. Leave for 5 minutes, then drain and toss the beans and noodles with some of the dressing.

Heat a ridged griddle pan until it is smoking. Place the tuna steaks on the griddle and sear for 1–2 minutes on each side. Remove and immediately slice thinly. Add the tuna, tomatoes, eggs, olives and basil to the beans and noodles; add more dressing to taste.

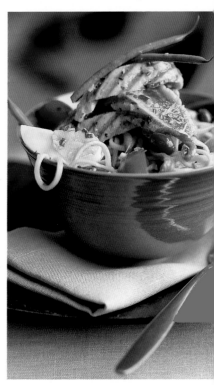

▲ *A perfect substitute for red meat, this tuna dish is low in fat and highly nutritious.*

hormone regulators

Plant oils containing gamma linolenic acid, or GLA, can ease premenstrual symptoms such as breast tenderness and cramping. Supplements are available in capsule or oil form.

balancing evening primrose

Gamma linolenic acid is an essential fatty acid that aids the production of prostaglandins. These are substances that help to maintain the body's hormonal balance and control the release of the sex hormones, oestrogen and testosterone. Probably the most common source of gamma linolenic acid is evening primrose oil. Taken over time, it has been shown to reduce a range of PMS symptoms, from breast tenderness to joint aches and skin complaints. It also helps to decrease the blood-clotting that can cause cramping. You will begin to feel the benefits of taking evening primrose oil supplements from one to three months after starting. Ask your medical practitioner about dosage.

borage oil

Also called starflower oil, borage oil is the richest source of gamma linolenic acid found in nature, at 22–5 per cent. This proportion is twice that of evening primrose oil. Borage supplements are often combined with evening primrose oil or flax oil, which also contains omega essential fatty acids. For the highest quality, look for capsules of cold-pressed, organic oil.

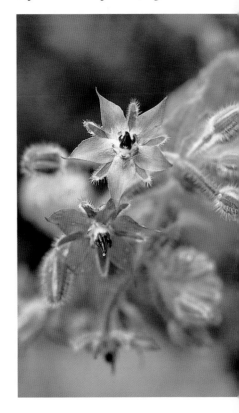

▸ *The borage plant yields an oil that, taken regularly, can help to balance hormones.*

162 vital vitamins C & E

Ensuring that you consume enough vitamins C and E by eating fresh fruits and vegetables will help relieve many PMS conditions. You can use supplements to top up your levels.

easing E

An essential fat-soluble substance, vitamin E is said to ease tenderness in the breasts and decrease the size of fibrous breast lumps before a period. Vitamin E is found in many types of foods, including nuts, seeds such as sunflower and pumpkin, cold-pressed oils, vegetables, spinach, whole grains, wheatgerm oil, asparagus, avocado, beef, seafood and carrots.

For PMS, it may be beneficial to increase the vitamin E in your diet with a daily supplement. Ask your medical practitioner for advice.

get your Cs

A shortage of vitamin C can result in water retention, a lack of energy and poor digestion, so it is a good idea to ensure that you are getting enough prior to and during your period. Also known as ascorbic acid, this vitamin assists with tissue growth, the healing of wounds and burns and the prevention of blood-clotting. Good food sources of vitamin C include fresh berries, citrus fruits, green leafy vegetables, guavas, tomatoes, melons and peppers. Daily supplements of 500–1,000mg may help to ease the symptoms of PMS.

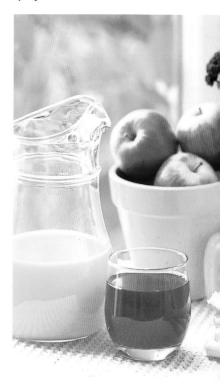

▸ *Citrus fruits and apples are rich sources of vitamin C. Eat whole or drink their juices.*

163 vitamin B6

Eating food containing a selection of B group vitamins is essential for cell growth, and vitamin B6 in particular may help alleviate many premenstrual symptoms.

Research has shown that vitamin B6 (pyridoxine) helps to balance female hormones and fight depression. The foods containing this vitamin include chicken, fish, liver, kidneys, eggs, walnuts and carrots. B group vitamins work best when taken together as a complex, and taking supplements of 50–100mg per day may help alleviate PMS symptoms. Be careful not to take in excess of 200mg, as this can cause reactions such as numbness and tingling in the feet and hands.

▼ *Like all fish, swordfish steaks contain vitamin B6, and are delicious when grilled.*

swordfish steaks
Serves 4
4 swordfish steaks, 175g/6oz each
60ml/4 tbsp extra virgin olive oil
juice of 1 lemon
30ml/2 tbsp chopped fresh parsley
salt and ground black pepper

Lay the swordfish in a shallow dish. Mix the remaining ingredients and pour over the steaks. Cover and leave to marinate for 10 minutes. Pat the fish dry with kitchen paper and grill for 2–3 minutes each side until just cooked through but still juicy. Serve with a rocket (arugula) salad.

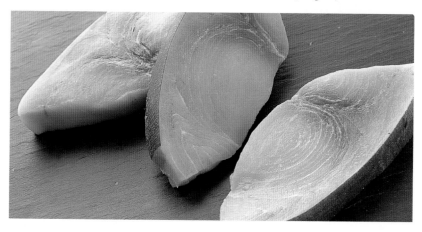

craving reducer

Magnesium has been shown to reduce cravings for sugar and chocolate. It can also reduce breast tenderness and migraine, two premenstrual symptoms that are suffered by many women.

beneficial mineral

Not only does it reduce the craving for sweets, the mineral magnesium also provides an effective boost to energy levels when you need it most. Magnesium deficiency can lead to tiredness and irritability. It also helps control blood pressure and keeps the heart muscle toned, and it works to help the body absorb calcium, an important mineral for cell function and bone formation.

Recent research in the USA has suggested that magnesium may also play a part in preventing migraines. In the studies, half the women who suffered from menstrual migraine were shown to have a magnesium deficiency at the time of the onset of their headaches.

getting enough

To consume magnesium in your premenstrual diet, choose from a wide selection of magnesium-rich foods, including dairy products, fish, legumes, apples, apricots, avocados, bananas, whole grain cereals, nuts and dark green vegetables. Cocoa is also a source of magnesium, which may be a reason for craving chocolate at this time if there is a deficiency. The recommended supplement dosage is 300–500mg per day, taken only when symptoms are present. Ask your medical practitioner for advice.

▲ *Dark green vegetables such as broccoli are good sources of magnesium.*

To alleviate cramps,

try taking the amino acid

DL phenylalanine –

ask your medical practitioner

about a suitable dosage

of the supplement.

166 natural diuretics

One of the most aggravating and uncomfortable premenstrual symptoms is water retention, which also triggers other PMS complaints. Herbs and supplements that have a diuretic effect can help.

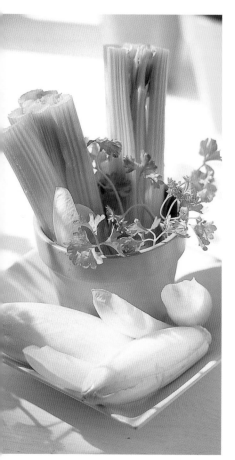

▲ Parsley, celery and chicory leaves have a natural diuretic effect on the system.

water weight

Many women experience significant weight gain in the days before a period, due to water retention. A whole host of other symptoms may also stem from it, from swollen breasts and limbs, to dizziness caused by the accumulation of water in the inner ear. Water retention can cause headaches and stuffy sinuses, due to pressure building in the skull, and it is also the cause of premenstrual backaches, stiff muscles and abdominal bloating.

herbal supplements

While there is no way to eradicate water retention totally, it is possible to get temporary relief from herbs and supplements. Chewing parsley or celery leaves can help, as can eating asparagus, and there are many other safe and natural herbal diuretics that are very effective at easing symptoms.

Tablet formulas and tinctures may include any of the following herbs, alone or in combination: boldo, *Uva ursi*, dandelion, juniper, celery and parsley. They are available from most chemists and health food shops. Use them only while symptoms are present.

asparagus with lemon sauce

Served here with a tangy lemon and egg sauce, asparagus is also delicious on its own dipped in melted butter.

Serves 4
675g/1½lb asparagus, tough ends
    removed, tied in a bundle
15ml/1 tbsp cornflour (cornstarch)
about 10ml/2 tsp sugar
2 egg yolks
juice of 1½ lemons

Cook the bundle of asparagus in plenty of salted boiling water for 7–10 minutes. Drain well, reserving 200m/7fl oz/scant 1 cup of the cooking liquid. Arrange the cooked asparagus in a serving dish.

To make the sauce, blend the cornflour with the cooled, reserved cooking liquid and place in a small pan. Bring to the boil, stirring constantly, and cook over a gentle heat until the sauce thickens slightly. Stir in the sugar, then remove the pan from the heat and allow to cool slightly. Beat the egg yolks with the lemon juice and stir gradually into the cooled sauce. Cook over a very low heat, stirring constantly, until the sauce is fairly thick. Be careful not to overheat the sauce or it may curdle. As soon as the sauce has thickened, remove the pan from the heat and continue stirring for 1 minute. Add salt or sugar to taste. Allow the sauce to cool slightly. Stir the cooled sauce, then pour a little over the asparagus. Cover and chill for at least 2 hours before serving the vegetables with the rest of the sauce.

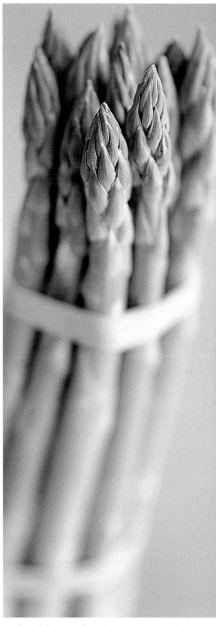

▲ *A well-known diuretic, asparagus makes a good seasonal choice for sufferers of pre-menstrual water retention.*

herbal migraine easers

Unfortunately, headaches and migraines are ailments that are very commonly associated with women's monthly cycles. But herbal remedies may relieve and even work to prevent them.

With any type of headache, taking a remedy at the first warning sign gives the best results. This is especially crucial with migraines, which can be heralded by symptoms including visual disturbances, a sharp ache at one side of the head, nausea and sensitivity to light, sound and smells.

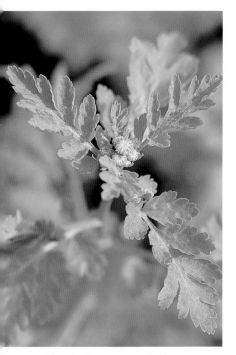

▲ *Feverfew is recommended by many healthcare advisers as a migraine remedy.*

feverfew relief

A member of the daisy family, feverfew is a well known natural remedy for headaches and migraines. Take it in the days before your period for prevention, and as early as possible during an attack.

butterbur

Taken regularly, butterbur is said to reduce the occurrence of migraines by about 60 per cent. Clinical trials show that the attacks that occur are less severe, and also of shorter duration. Like feverfew, it is available from health food stores and internet sites. Ask your healthcare practitioner for the correct dosage.

rosemary tisane

Rosemary clears the head and eases depression, improving the circulation and relieving headaches. For a pleasant-tasting, invigorating tea, seep one or two small fresh sprigs in 250ml/8fl oz/1 cup boiling water for about 5 minutes.

digestive aids

The days leading up to a period may be beset with digestive problems, from uncomfortable bloating and gassiness, to indigestion and nausea. Natural remedies can help to calm the digestion.

peppermint cure

One of the best and most readily available remedies for digestive upsets is peppermint. Its cooling sensation eliminates abdominal cramps, nausea, gas, bloating and spastic colon. For a digestive after a meal, make a tea from fresh or dried leaves by steeping in boiling water for 5 minutes; or add 1–2 drops peppermint oil to a glass of cold or hot water.

Oil of peppermint capsules are ideal if you are at work or out of the house. Spearmint, with its milder taste, is also beneficial, and can be used in the same way as peppermint. Chewing sugar-free, strong mint gum can also be beneficial.

comforting ginger

Used for thousands of years in China, ginger is very effective in soothing irritation of the intestinal membranes and aiding digestion. To use fresh ginger, place two or three thin slices of root ginger in a cup. Pour on boiling water and steep for 5 minutes. Add a teaspoon of honey to sweeten if desired, and drink. Powdered ginger may also be used.

lemon balm tea

An easy garden herb, lemon balm is helpful for indigestion and headaches and has a gentle sedative effect. Put 30ml/2 tbsp freshly gathered leaves into a pot and pour in 600ml/1 pint/ 2½ cups boiling water. Steep for 10 minutes then strain. Drink one cup three times a day.

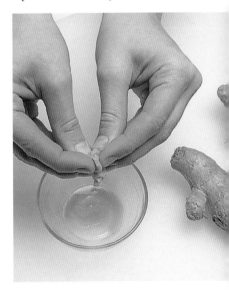

▲ *Fresh ginger slices can be infused in boiling water to make a delicious, fragrant digestive that brings instant relief.*

169 natural progesterone

Wild yam extract has been used for centuries in many cultures for its natural progesterone content. It can be used to treat a whole host of ailments, including premenstrual symptoms.

hormone imbalance

As the body ages, its production of progesterone – a hormone produced by the ovaries and also, to a lesser extent, by the adrenal glands – declines dramatically, leading to hormonal imbalances caused by an excess of oestrogen. These imbalances can lead to increased premenstrual symptoms, including water retention, variations in blood sugar levels (leading to mood and energy dips), depression and sleep disturbances.

wild yam extract

Natural progesterone creams made from plants such as wild yam can help normalize blood sugar levels, help the body use fat for energy, and clear up premenstrual acne and skin redness. They also have a natural diuretic and anti-depressant effect, and have been said to help prevent breast and endometrial cancers.

Progesterone cream is applied by rubbing it into the soft skin on the inner thigh, upper inner arm, chest or behind the knees. For PMS symptoms, 2.5ml/½ tsp is normally used twice daily for 21 days, stopping for seven days at the beginning of your cycle. Ask your healthcare practitioner for more information.

◀ *Progesterone cream is rubbed into the skin at soft tissue spots, where it is easily absorbed by the body.*

170 protective calcium

Calcium is an essential nutrient for women; it has been shown to be helpful in preventing and relieving premenstrual symptoms, and is important in the prevention of osteoporosis.

multiple relief

According to recent research, taking adequate calcium can help to reduce the physical and emotional effects of PMS by up to 50 per cent. Depression, mood swings, breast tenderness and abdominal and leg cramps may be relieved by ensuring that you eat enough foods containing calcium. Few people actually hit the recommended target of 1,000mg of calcium per day; some estimates indicate that the average woman manages only 500–700mg a day. So a supplement may be beneficial.

daily dose

Doctors recommend that women of child-bearing age should try to eat from a selection of dairy products such as milk, yogurt and cheese, and should also eat leafy green vegetables such as spinach, not just when PMS symptoms are present, but at all times of the month.

Try to work out how much calcium you get through your diet. If you think you have a shortfall, it may be a good idea to boost the amount to 1,000–1,200mg by taking a daily supplement of calcium carbonate.

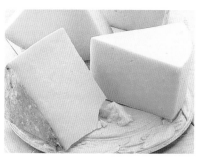

▲ *Cheese provides a concentrated amount of calcium. Choose low-fat varieties.*

▸ *Drinking semi-skimmed or skimmed milk is a good way to top up your calcium level.*

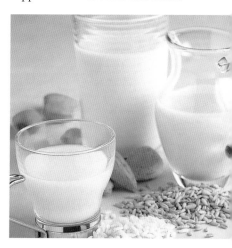

171 yoga for PMS

Excellent exercises at any time of the month, certain yoga postures – or *asanas* – can help to alleviate symptoms such as cramps, irregularity, backache, muscle ache and emotional tension.

wide-angled seated pose

On one or two folded blankets, sit with your back straight against a wall and arms at your sides. Spread your legs apart, as wide as possible. Keep the fronts of the legs facing the ceiling and the feet upright. Straighten the knees, then pull the thigh muscles back towards the groin. Draw up the trunk to extend the spine and open up the chest. Be sure to breathe evenly throughout. Stay in this position for 2–3 minutes, then release.

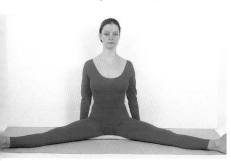

CAUTION:
You should not practise yoga poses during menstruation because they may interfere with the natural flow of blood.

half-lotus forward bend

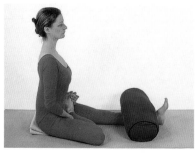

1 On a folded blanket, sit with your back straight and shoulders relaxed, with arms at your sides. Bend the right leg and place the foot on top of the left thigh, in the groin. Place a bolster on the left shin.

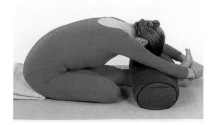

2 Bend forward and hold the left foot, resting your head on the bolster. Stay in this position for 30–40 seconds, then repeat on the other side.

172 aerobics for stress

When you're feeling anxious or down in the days before your period, doing an aerobic activity of your choice is one of the best ways to relieve stress and lift depression.

PMS specialists maintain that aerobic exercise, which raises the heart rate and is fuelled by oxygen, is essential for staying mentally and physically healthy, especially if you become frustrated, irritated and angry during the last two weeks of your cycle.

You need not attend a formal aerobics class: any activity that works up a sweat is aerobic. If you work sitting in an office all day, running up and down the stairs for a few minutes will make you feel better. Walking all or part of the way to and from work also helps you to wind down. Our bodies were designed to move, not to sit at a desk all day. Exercise uses up the hormone adrenaline that is produced when we become tense.

slow steps

If you have not exercised for a while, you may want to start by taking a leisurely 20-minute stroll during your lunch break, or getting out your bicycle after dinner and taking a tour of the neighbourhood with a friend. These gentle activities are a good choice when PMS symptoms such as tender breasts and cramps occur.

On the days that you feel more vigorous – possibly around ovulation, about 14 days before your period begins – tennis, badminton, dancing, jogging and running can all release tension. Whichever exercise you choose, aim to do a session of about 30 minutes at least three times a week.

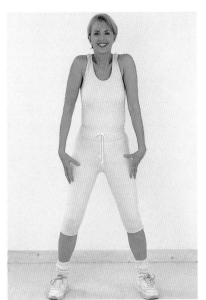

◀ Stretching the muscles before aerobic activity warms them and prevents injury.

173 Pilates treatment

Pilates is a system of exercise that aids muscle flexibility. It tones the girdle of muscles in the abdomen, strengthening the back and lessening the incidence of premenstrual backache.

the method

The Pilates Method was developed by Joseph Pilates over 70 years ago, and many variations of the exercise system have evolved since. Some forms are performed on specially designed exercise equipment, but many are carried out on the floor, using only a simple mat.

Using a series of controlled movements and breathing, Pilates exercises are designed to strengthen the deep postural muscles, building a "girdle of muscles" around the torso that protects your back from injury, aches and pains. The gentle movement makes for a refreshing workout that tones the whole body, while also improving the circulation, respiratory and lymphatic systems.

rolling back

The following exercise is the perfect foil for PMS aches as it mobilizes and massages the back muscles and abdominals. Once you have practised the movement with your hands on the floor, try progressing on to rolling back. Keep the chin tucked into the chest and do not grip the neck. You may not roll back up on your first attempt, but keep practising!

▼ *Pilates strengthens abdominal muscles.*

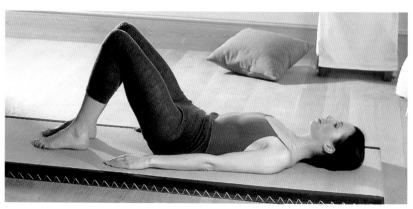

first position

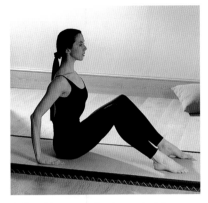

1 Sit with your spine in neutral, knees bent and feet on the floor. Place your hands near your hips. Inhaling deeply, draw your navel towards your spine. Lower your chin then, using your hands for support, start to roll down. Try to place each vertebra on the floor, one by one. To do this, tilt the pelvis and curve your spine into a C-shape.

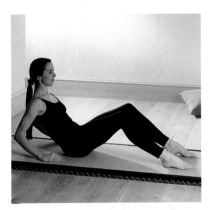

2 Once you have rolled down as far as you find comfortable, exhale and, using your core strength, return to your starting position. Pull up through the crown of your head to create a long spine, then repeat.

second position

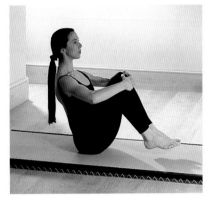

1 Sit upright with your spine in neutral. Lengthen up through the spine and imagine your head floating up to the ceiling. Place your feet flat on the floor and your hands just below your knees. Do not overgrip: keep elbows bent and your chest open. Take care not to tense or grip around your neck. Inhale as you tilt the pelvis to roll back.

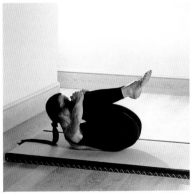

2 Curve the spine into a C-shape as you roll back, tucking in your chin and keeping your thighs close to your chest. As you exhale, use the abdominal muscles to pull you back up to the starting position.

174 muscle-fatigue relievers

Aching muscles – especially in the limbs – are a very common premenstrual symptom. These simple stretches will help to prevent the build-up of muscle tension.

calf stretch

Sit on the floor with one leg stretched out in front of you. Lean forward and grasp your foot with your hand. Pull your foot gently towards you, feeling the tightness in the calf. Hold for 30 seconds. If you cannot hold the foot in this position, try doing this stretch with the leg slightly bent. Repeat the exercise with the other leg.

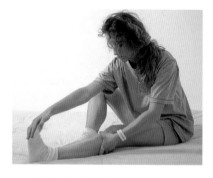

finger pulls

Squeeze a finger joint of one hand between the first finger and thumb of the other hand. Hold the base of the finger and then pull the finger gently, sliding your grip up to the top in a continuous movement. Repeat the exercise with all the fingers and thumbs of each hand.

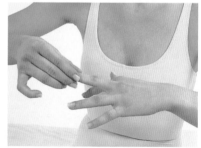

hamstring stretch

Lie down flat on the floor or exercise mat. Raise one leg and bend the other knee. Stretch the muscle in the raised leg by pulling it gently towards your chest. Hold for 20 seconds. Relax, then repeat with the other leg.

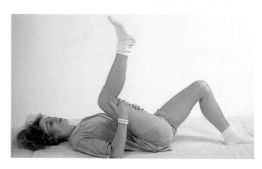

175 abdominal tension easer

Premenstrual emotional stress can lead to tension being stored in the abdominal area. These two exercises can help to loosen up the muscles, helping you to relax and breathe more deeply.

sideways bends

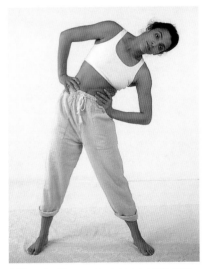

1 Stand with your feet apart and your hands on your hips. Bend over to one side, keeping your head in line with your torso – do not twist the body.

2 Slowly return to an upright position, then bend to the other side. Repeat on each side eight times. Do not bend further than is comfortable. Your flexibility should improve as you get used to the movement.

abdominal moves

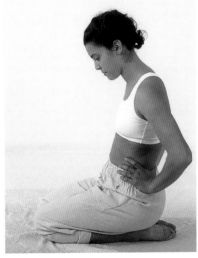

1 Sit cross-legged or kneel in a comfortable position, and place your hands on your waist or thighs. Let your breath out completely.

2 Without inhaling, pull in your abdomen as far as you can, then let it "snap" in and out up to five times before you take a breath. Relax for a few moments, then repeat the sequence three times.

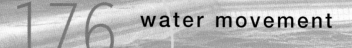

Use the support of comforting water to stretch fatigued muscles and tissues before your period – try swimming, aqua aerobics or water jogging.

177

pine & rosemary rub

Premenstrual tension can leave your neck and back aching and sore. This refreshing mixture, used in conjunction with massage from your partner or a friend, will bring you lasting relief.

Good for muscular aches and stiffness, marjoram and rosemary are both effective treatments, while invigorating oil of pine seeps deep into muscle tissue to provide relief from pain; it also relieves fatigue. You can ask your partner to massage the oil into tense areas, or use self-massage to work it into your neck and upper back.

pine, rosemary and marjoram rub

15ml/1 tbsp safflower, wheatgerm, jojoba or other carrier oil
1 drop pine essential oil
2 drops rosemary essential oil
2 drops marjoram essential oil

Wash and dry your hands, and make sure that the utensils are clean and dry. Measure the carrier oil into a small bowl. Add the pine, rosemary and marjoram oils, one drop at a time. Mix gently with a clean cocktail stick (toothpick).

> **CAUTION:**
> If you have sensitive skin, make a test mix with just one drop of essential oil to 20ml/4 tsp carrier oil and apply to a small area of skin before using for a full massage.

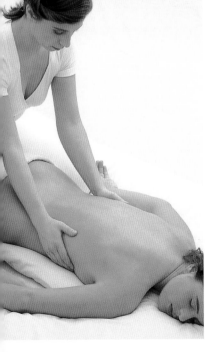

◀ A relaxing and deep back rub using an essential oil mixture will calm frayed nerves as well as soothing your body.

178 hormone-balancing oil

An increase of premenstrual oestrogen can lead to a range of complaints. This relaxing bath mix uses essences that may help to normalize hormonal secretions, easing the onset of symptoms.

Renowned for their beneficial effect on the female reproductive system, clary sage and naiouli relax cramped muscles, while cypress helps ovarian problems. Use this bath oil for 10–12 days before the start of your period.

clary sage, naiouli and cypress bath
15ml/1 tbsp almond or other
    carrier oil
1 drop clary sage essential oil
2 drops naiouli essential oil
1 drop cypress essential oil

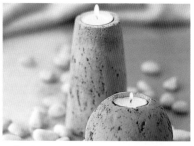

▲ *Setting the mood by lighting candles can help bring you into a state of relaxing calm.*

Run a very warm bath, but don't make the water too hot. Add the essential oils to the carrier oil in a small bowl and mix. Pour into the bath and swirl the water to distribute the oil. You may want to light candles and play soft music to help you wind down. Climb in and relax for not more than 15–20 minutes.

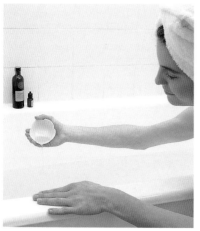

▲ *Breathe deeply to experience the full healing effect of the essential oils.*

CAUTION:
Clary sage should not be used if you suspect you may be pregnant. Extensive usage can cause problems with those taking the contraceptive pill or hormone replacement therapy (HRT).

179 crampbark compress

Sharp abdominal pain just before and during periods is due to the contraction of the womb muscles, which reduces blood flow. This hot compress acts to increase blood circulation.

pain-relieving abdomen compress
Crampbark is a herb that works to reduce spasm in the muscles, while rosemary, which is commonly grown in domestic gardens, is a circulatory stimulant that is particularly effective for treating conditions of the womb and the head.

Combining the fresh or dried herbs with the action of heat makes this compress an effective alternative to taking analgesic drugs, providing immediate relief from abdominal pain with no side effects.

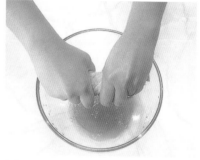

2 Soak a clean cotton cloth or cotton bandage in the liquid. Wring out when the cloth or bandage is cool enough to handle.

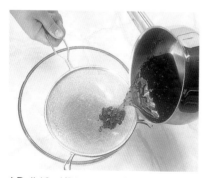

1 Boil 10ml/2 tsp crampbark in 600ml/1 pint/2½ cups water for 10–15 minutes. Add 10ml/2 tsp dried rosemary, or 15ml/3 tsp fresh leaves. Leave for 15 minutes, then strain.

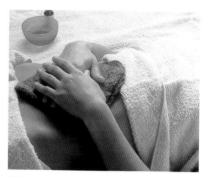

3 Lie down in a comfortable, warm place, lay the hot compress over your abdomen and relax for at least 10 minutes while the soothing properties of the herbs take effect.

180 soothing head massage

Aromatherapy massage can help overcome a debilitating migraine brought on by hormonal changes. To treat a migraine at other times, omit the clary sage if you think you may be pregnant.

early action

Many women experience an "aura", seeing a light halo around objects, the day before a migraine attack begins. Some sufferers have a heightened sensitivity to smell. At the earliest sign of a migraine, you can try using this aromatherapy treatment. Add 2 drops rosemary, 1 drop clary sage and 1 drop marjoram to 15ml/1 tbsp of a light carrier oil such as sweet almond or jojoba. Mix the oils together, then rub a small quantity of the oil between the fingers to warm it.

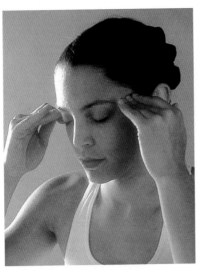 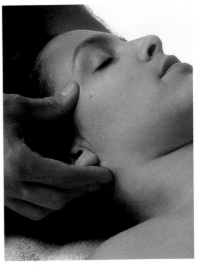

1 Self-massage can be effective. Begin by gently massaging the temples with the oil, using small circular movements. Move the fingers up to massage the forehead and then bring them back to the temples.

2 A gentle head massage from a partner can be even more beneficial. Ask them to massage a small amount of oil into your temples and forehead, then gently work into the hairline and the back of the neck.

181 menthol inhalation

Minor yet annoying respiratory and sinus problems are common PMS symptoms. An inhalation that uses natural menthol and purifying lemon can help you to breathe more easily.

During the week leading up to their period, many women experience an annoying catarrh at the back of their throat, or suffer from stuffed sinuses. The vocal cords may also become tight, making life more difficult for speakers and singers. As well as drinking plenty of water, using a steam inhalation moistens and warms the membranes; adding essential oils helps to open and relax the airways. Eucalyptus is particularly helpful for the sinuses, chest and nose, and lemon has a cleansing effect.

easy breathing inhalation
Boil a kettle and pour the hot water into a wide bowl. Add 3 drops eucalyptus essential oil and 2 drops lemon essential oil; you could try using 1–2 more drops for a stronger effect. Tilt your head over the bowl and inhale deeply for 2–3 minutes. Keep a comfortable distance away from the steam as it can burn the skin.

▾ *Steam inhalations can be a fast and effective way to provide immediate relief from minor respiratory complaints.*

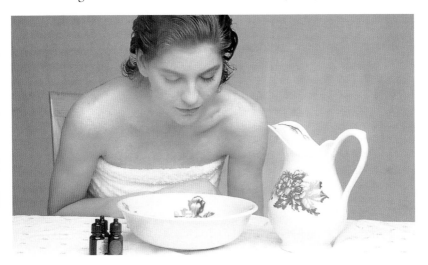

182 calming incenses & oils

Many people find the burning of incense resin or essential oils very soothing during times of premenstrual stress, either when doing meditation or simply while relaxing.

frankincense and myrrh

Used for centuries in religious ceremonies and as a meditation aid, frankincense deepens and slows the breath. It dispels nervous tension and fear, and is useful for painful periods. Myrrh has also been used since ancient times; it has antiseptic and healing qualities that cleanse the air and calm the spirits. Add 2 drops frankincense and 2 drops myrrh essential oils to water in the bowl of an oil burner. Alternatively, burn nuggets of both resins in a charcoal burner, or use incense sticks.

orange, neroli and benzoin

Another calming combination to try is neroli, benzoin and orange peel. Neroli soothes the nerves with its hypnotic and euphoric effect, and can bestow a sense of peace during times of premenstrual tension, anxiety and low self-confidence. Benzoin is soothing for temporary emotional turbulence, such as that caused by pre-period mood swings. It helps you to let go of worries and quells feelings of depression. The addition of orange gives a lift to the senses and relieves exhaustion. For an aromatherapy mix, add 2 drops neroli, 2 drops benzoin and 2 drops orange essential oils to water in the bowl of an oil burner.

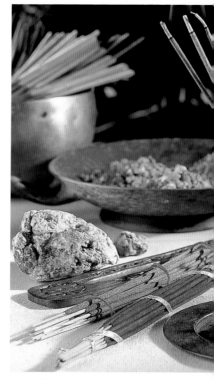

▲ *Burning frankincense and myrrh can help release tension and aid meditation.*

183 rose & jasmine soother

The days leading up to a period may be fraught with frustrated and angry feelings. This oil blend can help if you start to feel tense and critical of family, friends and colleagues.

The abdomen is the "seat of the emotions" – tension may build and be stored here, causing irritation, especially before menstruation. This calming abdominal rub can be used as a salve to calm frayed nerves. The beautiful scents of rose and jasmine are both uplifting and soothing to the nervous system.

rose and jasmine soother

In a bowl or bottle, add 3 drops of rose essential oil and 3 drops jasmine essential oil to 75ml/5 tbsp of carrier oil such as almond to make up a massage oil; stir or shake to disperse.

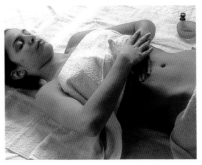

2 Move your hands in a clockwise direction, trying to keep the muscles relaxed the whole time. Breathe deeply to get the benefit of the scent.

ROSE

The rose has been prized throughout history for its restorative properties, including treatment of irregular and painful periods, headaches, insomnia, depression and stomach upsets of an emotional origin.

JASMINE

The strong smell of jasmine – which has been described as "the scent of angels" – is good for general PMS complaints and painful periods. It promotes feelings of optimism, euphoria and confidence.

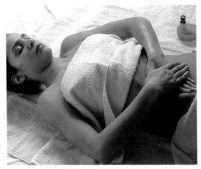

1 Using a little of the oil in your palms, slowly and firmly rub the abdomen with your hands.

The **chaste tree** berry has been known to ease general **PMS symptoms**. For best effect, take drops of the **tincture** two or three times daily during the week before **menstruation**.

185 lower back relaxer

The lumbar area of the back, where it curves towards the pelvis, is a common premenstrual hot spot. A massage from your partner will do much to alleviate discomfort and pain.

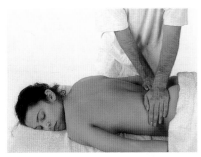

1 Find somewhere comfortable for your partner to lie for the treatment. Standing or kneeling to the side, place your hands on the opposite side of your partner's back and pull them toward you firmly. Work down the back to the base of the spine, always keeping in mind the comfort of the person you are massaging.

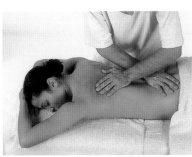

2 Overlap the hands to create an effect similar to bandaging, but ensure that you do this with a soothing, caressing motion. Because this can be a sensitive and painful area at this time of the month, ask your partner how hard she would like the pressure to be and adjust your movements as necessary.

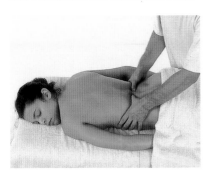

3 Using your thumbs, make circling movements over the lower back. Use a steady, even pressure, leaning with your body, but do not press on the spine because this might cause discomfort and pain. Continue this movement for approximately 5 minutes, then repeat step 2, but use lighter movements in order to end the massage.

186 therapies for legs & feet

Many women experience water retention and cramps during their cycle. Massage will help release water from cells in the thighs and legs, while acupressure can also ease these symptoms.

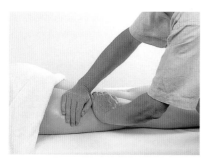

thigh and leg massage

1 In order to improve someone's circulation, warm a little massage oil in the palms of your hands, then apply to the legs. Place both hands on the thigh and stroke upward to the buttocks a few times. Use light but steady sweeping movements, hand-over-hand.

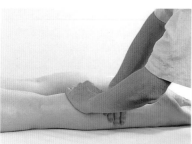

2 Move hands down to the lower leg and stroke up to the back of the knee a few times. Repeat steps 1 and 2 on the other leg, remembering always to stroke upward toward the heart.

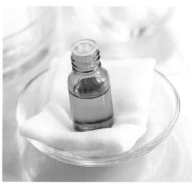

▲ Lemon oil is an excellent essential oil for reducing water retention. Use a little at first to check whether your skin is sensitive to it.

THERAPEUTIC OILS
The essential oil from the juniper berry has a diuretic effect, so for massage you can add 2 drops to 30ml/2 tbsp carrier oil. Other oils to try include grapefruit, geranium and lemon oil. Use citrus oils sparingly until you are sure that your skin is not sensitive to them.

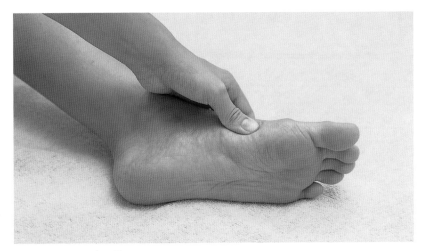

acupressure point for cramps

For cramps and digestive problems turn your right foot on its side. Use your right thumb to locate the pressure point one thumb-width down from the fall of the foot, close to the inner edge. This is Spleen 4. Press firmly (but not painfully) and hold for one minute. Release the pressure and pause for another minute, then repeat. Breathe deeply while pressing the point. Repeat on the left foot.

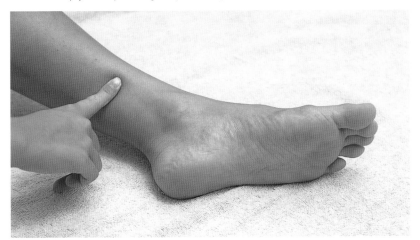

acupressure point for irregular periods and water retention

To ease these two common symptoms of PMS, turn your right lower leg on its side. Use your right index finger to find the pressure point four finger-widths up from the inner ankle bone, close to the side of the shinbone. This is Spleen 6. Press this point for one minute. Release for a few moments, then press again for another minute. Keep breathing as you press. Repeat the action on the left foot.

187 abdomen massage

A gentle massage from a partner or friend can help relieve premenstrual cramping and discomfort in the abdominal region. Do not use this massage after a heavy meal.

A drop or two of peppermint or spearmint oil added to a tablespoon of carrier oil – such as grapeseed or sunflower – will add a soothing, cool dimension to this massage. The essential oils of the mint family contain menthol, which is a natural digestive that can be helpful when used externally as well as internally.

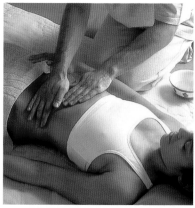

2 Adjust the depth of pressure to your partner's comfort level. If it is increased slowly and gradually, deeper pressure can be very relaxing, but you should not overdo it.

ABDOMINAL PAIN
Regular full-body massage using recommended essential oils, such as chamomile, clary sage, hops, lavender, marjoram, rose and rosemary, can help to alleviate period pains. However, severe pain should always be investigated by a medical practitioner, as it may indicate a gynaecological disorder.

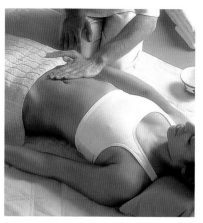

1 Rub a little massage oil into your hands to warm it. On the abdomen, use very slow circling movements in a clockwise direction, to aid the digestive process. Make sure your partner feels comfortable with this movement and is relaxed.

helpful homeopathy

Many women are prone to premenstrual mood swings and pain. Homeopathy treatments, whereby tiny amounts of plant, mineral or animal substances are taken, can help.

Homeopathy is a holistic therapy based on the principle of "like cures like". Formulated by Samuel Hahnemann in the 19th century, it works on the premise that infinitesimally small amounts of a substance which, in a healthy person, would produce symptoms of a particular complaint, will stimulate the immune system of a sufferer to combat that same complaint. A range of remedies, taken singly or together, can help ease PMS symptoms.

emotional rescue

Along with moodiness, some women are beset with symptoms of depression, anger and weepiness, even as much as a week or more before the flow begins. *Pulsatilla* is an excellent remedy if weeping and the feeling of neediness are prominent. *Sepia* can be used where there is anger and exhaustion, and can even lessen feelings of indifference to your family. For extreme symptoms of violent anger and jealousy, *Lachesis* is helpful.

▸ *Consult a qualified practitioner for advice on homeopathic treatments for PMS.*

period pain aid

For cramping pains that respond to warmth (a hot water bottle, for example) and make you want to curl up, *Mag phos* should provide some relief. For very severe pains with bad cramping, *Viburnum opulus* is a powerful painkiller.

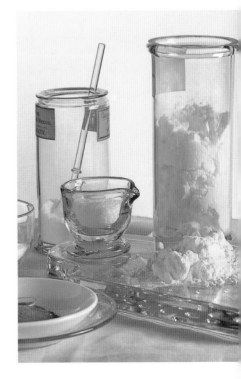

Find a quiet spot, and sit with your hands resting lightly on your lap.

Close your eyes and draw in a deep breath from the bottom of your lungs, counting to ten. Slowly release on another count of ten.

relieving reflexology

Reflexology works on the premise that reflex points on the feet, hands and head correspond to other areas of the body. It can help ease PMS symptoms such as cramps and aching breasts.

menstrual cramps

Applying pressure with the thumb and fingers to the areas marked on the feet in the photographs can provide relief for abdominal cramps around the time of menstruation.

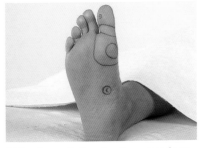

3 Finally, work the glands on one foot and repeat on the other.

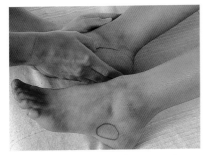

1 Work the lower spine for nerves to the uterus.

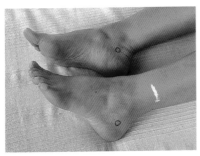

2 Next, work the uterus reflex on the sides of the heels.

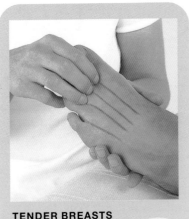

TENDER BREASTS
To soothe painful or tender breasts, fingerwalk up the "chest" area, marked on top of the foot, with three fingers together.

191 reiki PMS treatment

A quick and subtle treatment, reiki works on the premise that the practitioner helps the healing flow of energy in you, the recipient, assisting your own body and emotions to heal themselves.

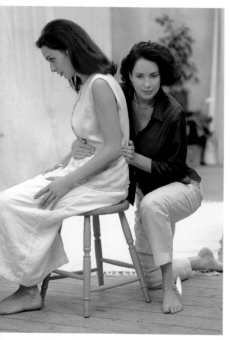

▲ *The reiki practitioner places hands directly on your body to direct energy flow.*

power over pain

Perhaps reiki's greatest gift is the empowerment of individuals to take responsibility for themselves and their own healing. Reiki energy can be so fast-acting, yet so subtle, that some ailments can fade away almost imperceptibly, together with the emotional triggers that may have been behind them. When considering reiki treatment for premenstrual symptoms, it is best to make an appointment with a qualified reiki practitioner. Many practitioners are happy to teach you self-treatment techniques. Some also practise "distance reiki" – a healing flow of energy sent to you without your having to be in the healer's presence.

menstrual pain

In reiki healing for menstrual pain, the practitioner will ask you to sit down or perhaps to stretch out on a sofa. She will then place one hand on your lower stomach and the other on the lower back, for relief from pain and cramping. This will lighten and relieve the surrounding area, including the thighs.

One philosophy associated with reiki treatment is that women can use this time to celebrate female unity and the expression of female energy, rather than view their pain as a purely negative thing.

192 balancing crystals

Period pain and menstrual cramps are often made worse by physical and emotional tension restricting the body's natural energy flow. Crystals can help to redress the balance.

mood-adjusting moonstones

In crystal therapy, moonstones, whether natural, tumbled or gem-polished, are said to be the ideal stones for women to wear, according to ancient Indian Ayurvedic texts. Moonstone is helpful in balancing and relaxing emotional states. It also has beneficial effects on all fluid systems in the body, and eases tension in the abdominal area.

A healing pattern of five moonstones amplifies the relaxing and healing potential of the stones. Place one moonstone at the top of your head, one on the front of each shoulder by the armpit and one resting on each hip.

chakra-opening opals

Dark opal has similar qualities to those of the moonstone, though it acts mainly on the first chakra – the energy centre that balances the sense of "self" – and the second chakra, the base of the sexual organs and the emotions, where it can often ease menstrual cramps in a very short time. Place a small piece of opal in a hip or trouser pocket.

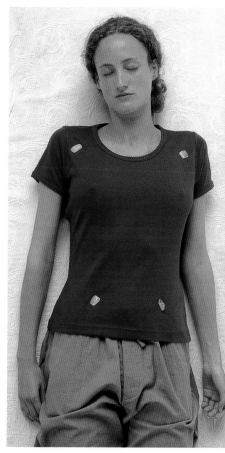

▲ *Moonstones and opals help to open up the chakras, assisting emotional healing.*

193 dealing with moodiness

Many women become susceptible to mood swings and depression in the week before a period, but there are a number of positive measures you can take to give yourself a lift.

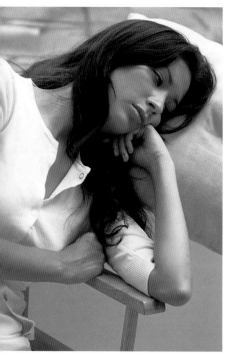

▲ *If you can control your thoughts, you can steer your mood into a more positive vein.*

take time out

You think you're having a great day, then suddenly someone says the wrong thing and you snap. From anger and frustration to anxiety and panic, hormones can play havoc with the moods and emotions. First of all, stop and remind yourself what time of the month it is, and give yourself a little slack. It's better not to take your frustrations out on others, so if you need a few minutes on your own, make your excuses and go for a walk, or sit and meditate in a quiet place. Take a deep breath and try to reach your "centre" – the true you beyond turbulent emotions or obsessive thoughts. But if you are feeling seriously depressed or out of control, talk to your doctor or a counsellor – don't suffer in silence.

make laughter essential

PMS can make some women feel stressed or unable to cope. One of the best ways of dealing with these feelings is to make sure you have a good laugh every day. Laughter raises the level of endorphins, the body's "feel good" substances. Sharing a few jokes with friends is a good way to dissipate negativity, as is watching a funny film or television show. Stepping back and laughing at your own dramas is excellent medicine.

Many women experience an increase in libido before or during their periods. Instead of letting the energy lead to frustration, you can use this time to explore your sexuality with your partner.

Emotions and sexual urges can run high from the time of ovulation through to your period. This provides a good opportunity to try new techniques and ways of lovemaking with your partner. You could start by giving each other an intimate massage, or sharing a bath. Perhaps you could share sexual thoughts and fantasies, then decide which ones to act out. Create a sensual atmosphere by lighting candles, sharing wine and shutting out the rest of the world.

▼ Intimacy can lead you both to explore your depth of feeling for each other.

beyond the physical

As well as reading books on sexual technique, it can be enlightening to explore different approaches to sex, such as the holistic view of love-making of Tantric philosophy. This school of thought evolved in ancient India and Tibet about 5,000 years ago. Today it is practised by those who want to enjoy greater intimacy of mind, body and spirit with their partner. Tantra sees a sexual relationship not only as the physical union of two people, but a re-enactment of the divine principle of union that governs the whole of existence.

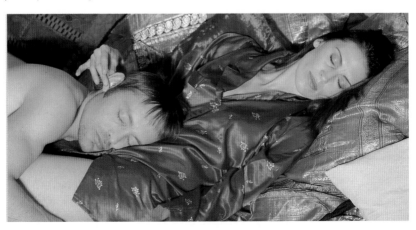

creative time out

For women of many cultures around the world, menstruation is seen as a time to celebrate their womanhood and the natural cycle of life, not as a time to be dreaded or ignored.

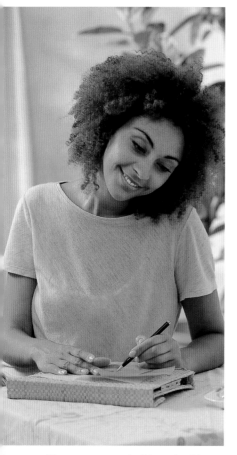

▲ *Many women use the "down time" in their natural cycles to reflect and create.*

a place away

Traditionally, among tribal peoples such as Native North Americans, a special menstrual hut was built so that a woman could go and be on her own to gather her thoughts, and find ideas through dreams and meditation. When she emerged from this "moontime", as it is sometimes called, it would be with songs, stories and insights into future endeavours. In such cultures it is believed that, just as the moon waxes and wanes, a woman reflects the changes in nature in her monthly cycle, and she is treasured for being this way.

meaningful moontime

You can make this time of every month a positive pathway to personal growth and change. By taking time to rest and reflect, instead of fighting the urge to slow down, you may be surprised by the clarity of the new ideas that surface. Indulge in your favourite pursuit or hobby, and give yourself room just to "be" with it – whether it is painting, music, cooking, astronomy, or devising a new system for your line of work.

196 soothing meditation

Meditation can help to bring body and mind into a state of harmony, allowing you to see your world in perspective. This meditation uses the clarity and depth of water imagery to focus the mind.

the well

You find yourself standing near the edge of a pond, looking down into the clear, cool water, gazing at goldfish, red and gold, black and silver, swimming so easily. . . gliding effortlessly in and out of the pondweed and around the lily pads. Your mind becomes deeply relaxed. You notice that the centre of the pond is very, very deep. It could be the top of a disused well. . . You take a silver coin and toss it into the very centre of the pond. . . then watch as it swivels down through the water. Ripples form, but you just watch the coin as it drifts and sinks, deeper and deeper through the clear water. . . Sometimes it seems to disappear as it turns on edge; at other times a face of the coin catches the sunlight and flashes through the water. . . twisting and turning on its way down. . .

Finally, it comes to rest at the bottom of the pond, lying on a cushion of soft brown mud. . . And you feel as still and undisturbed as the coin. . . as still, cool and motionless as the water, enjoying the feeling of inner peace and utter tranquillity.

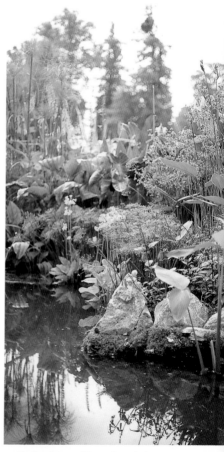

▲ Gazing into a still pond can help you to still your mind for meditation.

moon cycles

The moon has been linked with women and the female reproductive cycle from the earliest times. Most moon deities, such as the Greek Artemis and her Roman counterpart Diana, are female.

Many ancient civilizations venerated the moon because they saw how she influenced the germination and growth of crops, and how she also matched the average female menstrual cycle of 28–30 days. Some ancient cultures worshipped several moon goddesses, who represented the different phases of the moon. The Greeks, for example, honoured Artemis as the new moon, Selene as the full moon and Hecate as the waning and dark moon.

To understand your place in the fertility cycle of nature, it can help to study the moon lore of different cultures and see how these concepts can be related to the energy flow of your own monthly cycle.

female synchronicity
It is a well-known phenomenon that the menstrual cycles of women who live in close proximity to each other – whether flatmates, colleagues, mother and daughters, sisters or friends – tend to synchronize so that their periods start at the same time. This can happen surprisingly quickly, so if you start a new job or get a new flatmate, your menstrual start days may shift over one or two months. One theory is that the woman with the most healthy immune system leads.

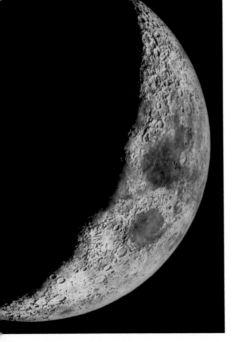

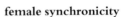
◂ *The moon and her cycles have always been linked with women's cycles, both physically and spiritually.*

planning ahead

By keeping a chart of premenstrual symptoms, both physical and emotional, you will be able to get an overview of the impact they have on your life, thus allowing you to plan ahead.

Apart from illustrating the rhythm of your life, compiling a chart will help you plan tasks for days of the month when you are feeling more energetic. It will help you to anticipate possible bouts of moodiness and frustration, and signal when you should start taking preventive supplements for these symptoms as well as maladies such as headaches and menstrual cramps.

	J	F	M	A	M	J	J	A	S	O	N	D
1												
2												
3												
4												
5												
6												
7												
8												
9												
10												
11												
12												
13												
14												
15												
16												
17												
18												
19												
20												
21												
22												
23												
24												
25												
26												
27												
28												
29												
30												
31												

Use this simple key to record symptoms, along with "M" for menstruation days.

D = Depression
T = Tearfulness
I = Irritability
S = Sleep disturbance
F = Fatigue
A = Abdominal cramps
H = Headache
J = Joint stiffness
B = Bloating
G = General aches/backache
C = Food cravings
W = Weight gain

sleep therapy

Especially during your period, which places special demands on your body, getting a good night's sleep is essential if you are to feel your best throughout the day.

setting the sleep scene

Make sure that your bedroom environment is quiet, pleasant, comfortable and airy. A woman's body temperature normally rises slightly before her period, so wear a lighter nightgown. If you are prone to premenstrual insomnia, try a sedative herbal infusion, such as chamomile or valerian tea, or a hot milky drink, an hour before going to bed. Fresh bedlinen and sprigs of fragrant lavender on your bedside table will help ease you into slumber.

calming mood

Sometimes it is difficult to sleep due to excessive emotions such as fear, depression or anxiety, caused by hormonal changes. Meditation techniques – such as surrounding yourself with a healing colour or visualizing a spiritual protector – can help quell your jumpy nerves. Try not to watch disturbing or violent television shows or read thrillers before going to sleep – these can enter your thought stream unawares and add to, or actually create, anxiety. Instead, read poetry or "light" stories, and listen to soothing music.

sweet dreams

Many women experience vivid and colourful dreams around their periods. Enjoy these by writing down the plots, along with inspiring images or ideas. Pay particular attention to people in your dreams: you could gain special insights about friends and family members, as telepathy can be strong at this time of the month.

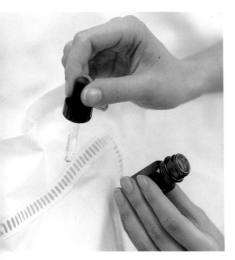

◄ *Scent your bedlinen with a few drops of soothing lavender essential oil.*

200 confidence boosters

PMS can make you very self-critical, and you may suffer from temporary low self-esteem. Reminding yourself of achievements and spending time with friends can serve to boost your confidence.

positive affirmations

Make a list of your achievements and attributes you are proud of, and stick it on a mirror or the refrigerator as a reminder of why you are lovable, competent, fun to be with and attractive. For example, your list could include affirmations such as: "I am a lovable person", "I am very good at painting or cooking", "My work colleagues hold me in great esteem", "I am a wonderful partner/mother/friend", "I am physically beautiful/have great legs/attractive eyes".

You can also remind yourself, "I may be feeling clumsy and lethargic at the moment, but this is natural and I accept it. In five days I will be my energetic self again."

enjoyable activities

Another way to increase your confidence when you're feeling low is to make time to do something you enjoy every day. Tell yourself that you are worth it, even if you are busy. Drop your chores, work or other responsibilities for an hour and do something you love doing – it is guaranteed to boost your spirits.

Make sure you also spend time talking with friends and family. Ask for the reassurance and physical contact – such as hugs – that you need. They will be happy to help out, and this will enable them to ask for support in turn when they need it.

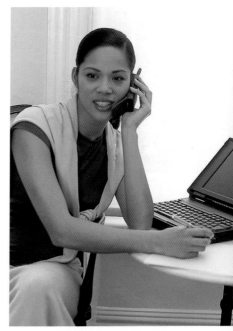

▲ Staying confident means keeping in touch with important people in your life.

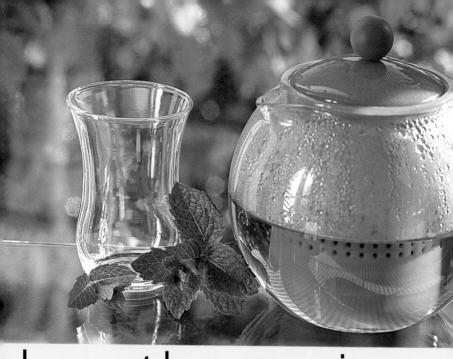

breathe easier

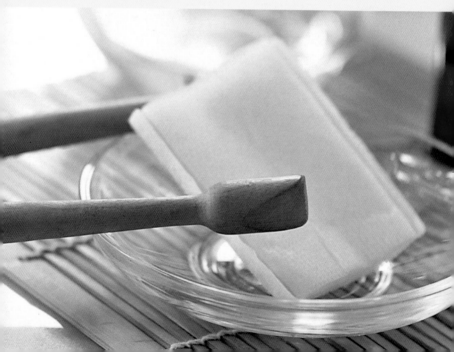

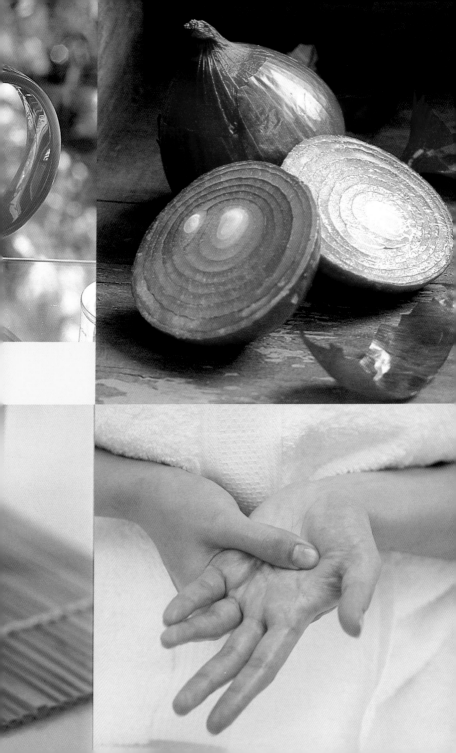

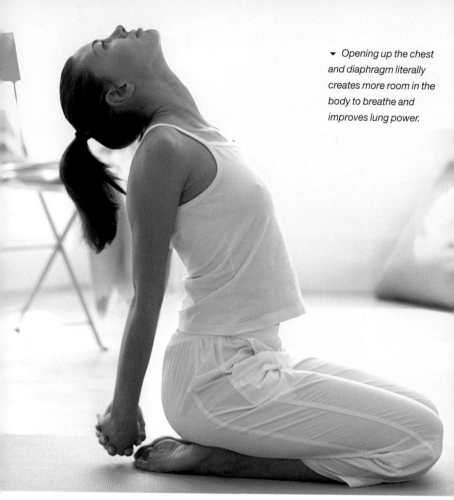

▾ Opening up the chest and diaphragm literally creates more room in the body to breathe and improves lung power.

a guide to better breathing

To breathe is to be alive. From the moment we take our first breath until we finally expire, breathing is what connects each and every one of us to life. It is estimated that we breathe in and out nearly 25,000 times a day, yet research estimates that only one in ten of us breathes correctly, and that most of us use only a fraction of our lung capacity.

And that is before we take into account the worrying increase in the occurrence of respiratory diseases and disorders, particularly those that are allergy-related.

This section contains 50 natural, drug-free treatments designed to help you breathe better. Some of these are aimed at specific complaints while others are targeted towards increasing lung capacity, building immunity and improving resistance to allergies and infections. However, first it is useful to understand how breathing works and how it influences our health.

the respiratory system

The human body can go without food for weeks and without water for days, but without oxygen we cannot survive for more than a few minutes. The body's breathing apparatus is known as the respiratory system and, together with the heart and blood supply, is probably the most important system in the body. When working properly it extracts the oxygen from the air that we need to live and discharges carbon dioxide waste from the blood.

The respiratory system is made up of the ribcage, with its linking intercostal muscles, the diaphragm – a sheet of muscle between the chest and stomach – and the respiratory tract, which comprises the airways and lungs. When we breathe in the diaphragm contracts and moves down increasing the capacity of the chest cavity, and the muscles that link the ribs contract, pulling the ribs up and out. These two processes cause the lungs to expand. Air is drawn in through the nose where it is warmed and taken down into the lungs. When enough air has been inhaled (inspiration), the muscles and diaphragm relax, compressing the lungs, and the air is exhaled (expiration). Then the diaphragm contracts once more and the cycle

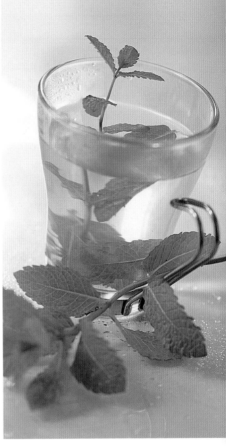

▲ Certain herbs, such as peppermint, can help to open up the airways.

begins again. After the air passes through the nose it enters the trachea (windpipe) and the bronchi, which are small airways that run through each lung. These bronchi become smaller and smaller, eventually taking the form of bronchioles, which end as tiny air sacs called alveoli. The alveoli are linked to blood capillaries that exchange oxygen and carbon dioxide at a very quick rate.

breathing rates

On average we take about 12 breaths per minute, according to the body's needs. If stressed, we tend to breathe at a faster rate, which can lead to muscle tension and eventually dizziness. Rapid breathing also occurs during strenuous exercise, an asthma attack or when frightened, because the body's need for oxygen increases. As the levels of oxygen and carbon dioxide return to normal, breathing resumes its usual slower rate. As we breathe normally and efficiently, the diaphragm contracts and becomes flat, increasing the space in the chest into which the lungs can expand. When the lungs are able to expand to their full capacity, all residual carbon dioxide is expelled and more oxygen can be inhaled.

breathing and health

The quality of our breathing affects our health in many different ways. Every cell in the body uses oxygen to extract the energy that is locked away in food, and our energy levels, mental powers, moods, creativity and emotional well-being all depend on the oxygen supply provided by our breathing. It is impossible to separate the health of our respiratory system from the rest of our lives, not only on a physical level, but also on mental and emotional levels.

Many ancient traditions have linked breathing with spiritual experience. The ancient Hebrews, for example, used the word "wind", the breath, in connection with the soul, and in India, "prana" or "spiritual breath" is seen as the life-force of the body's subtle energy system. So breathing affects our well-being at the level of mind, body and soul. It is our connection with the universe: trees and plants take in the carbon dioxide we exhale and replace it with life-giving oxygen in a cycle of integration and wholeness.

COMMON BREATHING PROBLEMS

The pressures of modern living have created an almost breathless culture. As we struggle to keep up with the fast pace of life, we become tense and anxious. This creates shallow and restricted breathing patterns, which lead to a tendency to over-breathe as we gulp in mouthfuls of air to compensate.

Furthermore, a variety of disorders – including physical injury, poor posture, infections, viruses, allergies and chronic disease – can disrupt and endanger the normal breathing process. Most breathing disorders are made worse by environmental pollution, or even by what we eat and drink, and in the case of allergies these can be the sole cause. Cigarette smoke also causes breathing problems, increasing the incidence of serious diseases such as lung cancer and emphysema.

Other disorders, ranging from the common cold, bronchitis and pleurisy to life-threatening conditions such as pneumonia and TB, are the result of bacterial or viral infections, which are made more likely by a weak immune system.

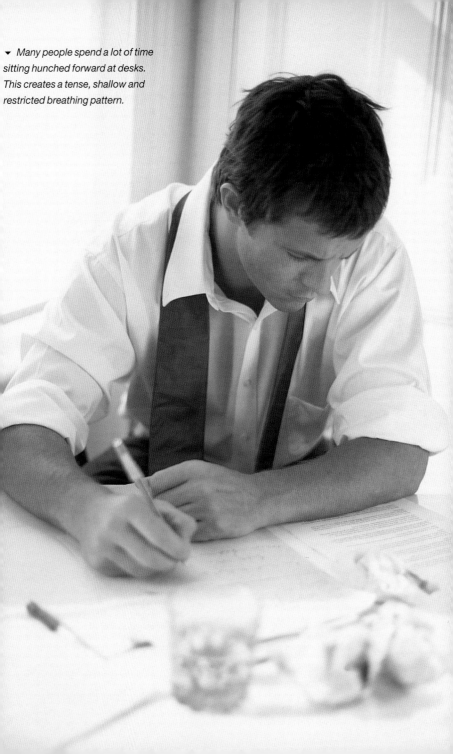

▼ *Many people spend a lot of time sitting hunched forward at desks. This creates a tense, shallow and restricted breathing pattern.*

breathing therapies

Whether our breathing problems are related to chronic asthma or bronchitis, to allergies such as hay fever and rhinitis,or the common cold, or even to poor posture, there are countless ways that we can improve our breathing and therefore the quality of our lives. The following pages present 50 natural, drug-free methods, some of which offer short-term quick-fix solutions, while others take a longer-term view. All, however, are based on holistic principles, recognizing that good health is achieved when mind, body and soul are balanced and in harmony.

The respiratory treatments that appear in this section are drawn from a variety of natural healing traditions, and include methods to re-educate our breathing as well as remedies and exercises that will rebalance, calm and strengthen it. Whatever the cause of your breathing difficulties, you are sure to find something here that works for you – in both the short and long term. You may try individual remedies or combine several that look as if they hold the key to your particular problem.

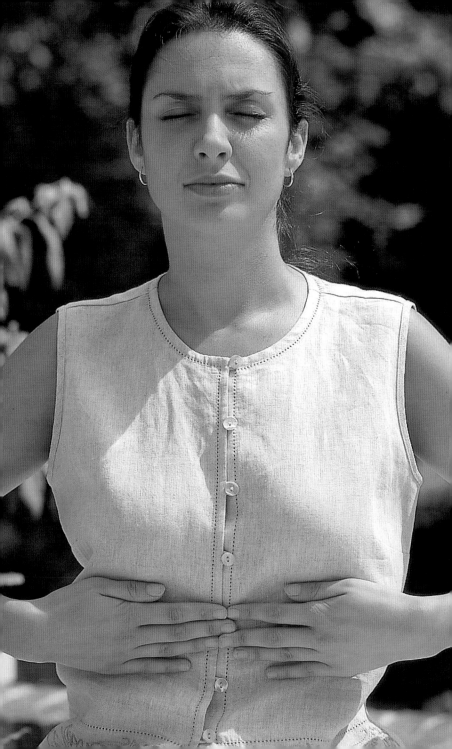

Buteyko method

Konstantin Buteyko (1923–2003), a Russian doctor, pioneered a theory and method of breathing that claims to be one of the most effective natural treatments for asthma and breathing disorders.

According to Buteyko, many breathing problems and disorders are linked to over-breathing, or hyperventilation, which causes an excessive reduction in the body's levels of carbon dioxide (CO_2).

health and carbon dioxide

Carbon dioxide is not only found in the atmosphere, but also in the alveoli (air sacs) in our lungs. Low levels of CO_2 in the body cause blood vessels to spasm (as happens in an asthma attack) so that oxygen is not properly absorbed by the body's tissues and vital organs. CO_2 is also involved in

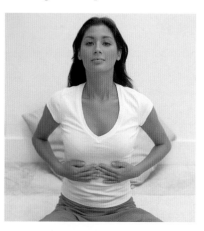

regulating the body's pH balance; insufficient CO_2 shifts the body towards alkalinity, which in turn has a weakening effect on the immune system, making it much more susceptible to viruses and allergies.

the Buteyko test

It is possible to measure your CO_2 level: breathe out, hold your nose and then count in seconds until you need to breathe in. A count of 60 corresponds to a level of 6.5 per cent CO_2 in the lungs and perfect health; between 40–50 is good, less than 30 indicates health problems, and if you have severe to moderate asthma, you may not be able to hold for more than 5–10 seconds.

self-help measure

Try to make an effort to breathe only through your nose, if possible. Buteyko practitioners claim that this practice alone can reduce asthma symptoms by up to 50 per cent.

◄ *The Buteyko method is based on retraining our breathing so that we take a longer pause at the end of the out-breath.*

202 alternate nostril breathing

When our breathing is calm and steady we are more able to think clearly. Calming and regulating the breathing is one of the best methods for stress reduction and improving concentration.

Our emotional state is reflected by our breathing patterns. So, if we are feeling nervous or under strain, we may tend to hyperventilate (over-breathe) or to inhale very short and shallow breaths.

The yoga technique that is known as alternate nostril breathing is designed to calm the nervous system, as well as harmonize the left and right sides of the brain. This also helps to redress any imbalance between introvert and extrovert tendencies – between an overactive mind that is draining our physical energies and an overexcited nervous system that is making us confused and mentally exhausted. It will also help clear blocked sinuses, so have some tissues handy.

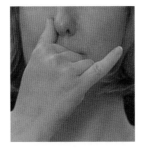

1 Two breaths form one round: do several rounds while sitting in an upright, comfortable position. Place your thumb at the base of your right nostril and pinch it closed. Breathe in through the left nostril.

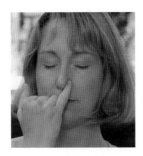

2 Relax your thumb and position your little finger at the base of the left nostril and pinch it closed. Breathe out through your right nostril. Your breathing will deepen slowly and naturally so don't force it.

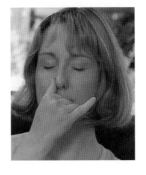

3 Now breathe in on the right, then close that nostril again and breathe out on the left. Continue to breathe slowly and steadily through alternate nostrils, using your thumb and finger to close the nostrils.

203 stretching & expanding

Expanding the chest enables the lungs to fill more efficiently with air, which will in turn bring extra oxygen to all the cells in the body, including the respiratory organs.

Chronic tension and anxiety can lead to restricted muscles, so that it becomes difficult to relax the diaphragm and breathe properly. Many asthmatics are tight around the diaphragm area, which exacerbates breathing difficulties. The following exercise is particularly good for asthma and other chest problems. When done on a regular basis, they will help improve breathing and blood flow to the chest muscles and lungs and help to open up the chest. First of all, stand with your feet hip-width apart, arms by your sides. Slowly taking a deep breath in, raise your arms out to the sides. Still breathing in, raise your arms up over your head, rising up on to your toes. Breathing out, drop your arms and return to standing. Then repeat this sequence twice more.

chest expansion

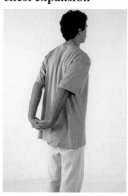 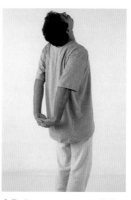 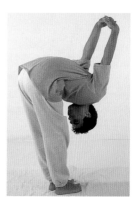

1 Stand with your feet hip-width apart and your knees slightly bent. Clasp your hands behind your back.

2 Raise your arms a little, leaning back slightly. Then lean forwards as far as possible, bending from the hips.

3 Raise your arms and keep them as high as is comfortable. Slowly straighten up, relax and repeat twice more.

204 making sounds

Singing, humming and playing a wind instrument are all excellent examples of how making sounds can help to strengthen our lungs and improve our breathing.

Playing a wind instrument (such as a flute or recorder) or singing is an effective way of improving your lung function and can really help counter hyperventilation. When you play a wind instrument, you are training yourself to control your breathing to produce the longest phrases. Singers also have to learn to control their breathing, so that they breathe in at an appropriate point in the song. If you feel too shy to sing in front of others, then practise when you are alone – in the shower or in the car, for example.

sound meditations

Combining sound with meditation is another way of improving lung capacity; it also has the advantage of quietening the mind and emotions. Try the following methods.

bee-breath meditation

This is a relaxing technique that is best done last thing at night to aid a good night's sleep.

Sit in an upright but relaxed position and close your eyes. Keeping your mouth closed, take a breath in. On the out-breath, start to make a humming sound, repeating the sound each time you breathe out. Keep your mind focused on the sound and let it become louder each time, so that you sound like a humming bee.

om-sound breathing

Sitting comfortably, inhale deeply and vocalize the sounds "ah", "oo" and "mm" as you exhale, joining them together to make the sound of "om". In the East, this is a sacred sound, the vibrations of which are said to heal and balance body, mind and spirit.

▼ Combining sound with meditation is a useful technique for calming our breathing.

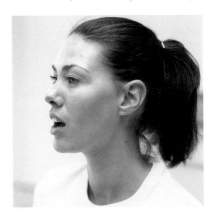

breathing exercises

To breathe is to be inspired. Breathing brings life-giving oxygen to the body and cleanses our system of impurities. Breathing exercises help to rebalance our breathing patterns.

Regulating your breathing helps you to feel calm and centred in body and mind. Breathing is also an excellent way of removing toxins from the body. Sitting still and breathing deeply after an indulgent night out, for instance, can help you feel get back on to an even keel. Try the simple cleansing exercise shown here. There are also many yoga exercises, known as "pranayama", that are based on working with the breath.

If you want to practise some serious breathing exercises it makes sense to seek out a teacher who can guide you until you are confident enough to exercise on your own. When practising anything more that a simple breathing routine a yoga mat will help your feet grip the floor and prevent your legs slipping. Light comfortable clothes are a good idea; some people prefer to practise in their underwear as this enables them to keep an eye on how their abdomen is moving. If this appeals, you'll need a warm room. The most important thing to remember is to always listen to what your body is telling you. If an exercise is hard work, try an easier option.

cleansing breath routine

This exercise has a powerful mucus-clearing action and so is ideal for those who suffer from allergies, a blocked nose or sinus trouble. It also strengthens the muscles of the abdomen, is good for a sluggish digestive system, and may even give your skin a healthy glow.

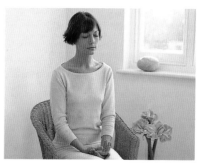

1 Sitting with your head up and your back straight, breathe out in a series of short, sharp exhalations through the nose. Tighten your stomach muscles and squeeze the air out of your lungs.

2 Relax your stomach muscles – you will automatically inhale. After the tenth in-breath, breathe out for as long as you can and try to empty the lungs. Take a few resting breaths and do another set.

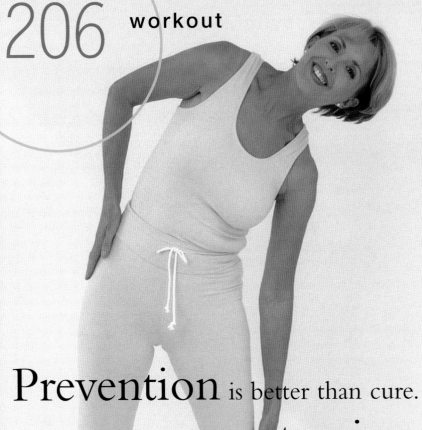

Prevention is better than cure. Aerobic exercise builds stamina, strengthens the immune system, and opens up the breathing. Try it and feel your body pulsate with life.

swimming

A session at your local pool provides one of the best types of exercise for strengthening the lungs, opening the chest and coordinating the breathing. It can help a wide range of breathing problems.

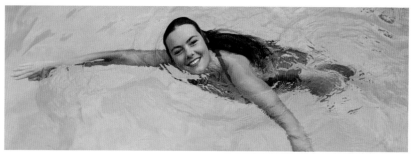

▲ *The benefits of swimming are well known. As well as being a good all-round form of exercise, it is especially helpful for regulating breathing disorders by reducing stress and tension and opening up the chest and diaphragm. Backstroke is particularly beneficial.*

Swimming is widely accepted as being a highly effective all-round form of exercise for the whole body. Its rhythmical actions encourage deeper breathing, increase lung capacity and improve the body's blood supply.

Regular sessions at the pool benefit the circulatory and respiratory systems and help to improve mobility in the joints and muscles, thus increasing muscular strength and tone. The immune system also gets a boost, making this form of exercise helpful for easing all kinds of conditions, including chronic breathing problems such as asthma.

Swimming can lessen the effects of stress and tension, which can produce tight or "held" patterns of breathing. If you have bronchitis or severe asthma, you may not be able to swim for long, but take it gently and you will gradually improve.

AQUA YOGA
Neatly uniting the benefits of yoga and swimming, aqua yoga combines slow stretching with breathing and relaxation techniques. Bodies feel virtually weightless in water, so more effective stretches can be achieved without the risk of strain.

yoga postures

Based on postures and breathwork, yoga can help with many breathing problems, as well as strengthening the immune system and building resistance to allergy and infection.

Yoga is both calming and energizing. Practised regularly it helps to increase stamina and flexibility, and also encourages the body to release patterns of tension and tightness. It does not matter how fit or flexible you are; the important thing while practising yoga (as with any form of exercise) is to work within your capabilities and not to strain or over-exert yourself in an attempt to achieve the "perfect" posture.

bridge pose

Lie flat on your back, arms by your sides. Bend your knees, feet hip-width apart, just in front of the buttocks. On an in-breath, lift your pelvis and raise your back so that you "stand" on your feet and shoulders. Breathe normally. On an out-breath, slowly lower yourself to the floor so that your buttocks reach the floor last.

simplified camel pose

Sit on your heels with your hands clasped behind you and breathe in. On the out-breath, drop your head back and raise your arms a little. Breathe for a few seconds, then return to an upright position on an out-breath. Repeat three or four times.

▼ *The "bridge pose" expands the ribcage and can be helpful in encouraging the expulsion of mucus.*

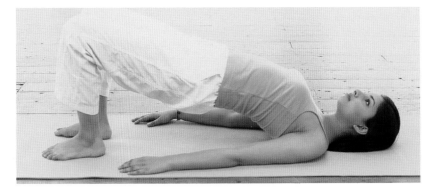

209 t'ai chi

In China, the non-combative martial arts system called t'ai chi is very much a part of daily life. Its gentle, meditative movements ease stress and help to deepen and regulate breathing.

The connection between breath, vital energy and consciousness is recognized by all the ancient spiritual traditions. In Taoist tradition, the breath is never held. Instead, absolute relaxation of the breath is cultivated, allowing it to become progressively smoother in its transition from yin (breathing in) to yang (breathing out) and back again.

breathing practice

Follow your breath in through your nose and down to the top of the throat. Be aware of all the sensations it generates, from the physical, to the energetic, to the emotional. As you breathe out, follow your breath back along this pathway, and relax and let go of everything you feel, allowing your energy to release fully. Continue to breathe along this pathway until you feel your breathing dropping lower, into the throat. Let your breathing become more relaxed and continuous (from in to out, without holding or stopping), following the breath as it naturally drops through the centreline of your body. Do not force the pace: it will only increase your level of internal tension and be counterproductive.

four-directional breathing

1 Stand with your feet apart and knees slightly bent. As you inhale, bring your hands, palms face-up, to chest height.

2 As you exhale, turn the palms to face away from you and extend your arms as if pushing something away.

1

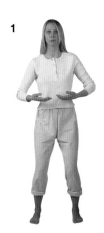

2

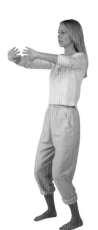

3 On the next inhalation, turn your palms back to face your body. Soften and relax your arms and draw them back in towards your chest.

4 Exhale, turning the palms out and extending your arms to your sides.

5 Inhale and bring your arms in towards your chest again.

6 On the next out-breath, turn your palms face-up and reach up towards the sky.

7 Inhale and let your arms descend, palms face-down.

8 As your hands and arms pass below your navel, begin breathing out and push down-wards with your hands, sending the energy towards the earth.

On the next inhalation, bring your hands up to begin a new cycle of four breaths. Repeat the sequence several times.

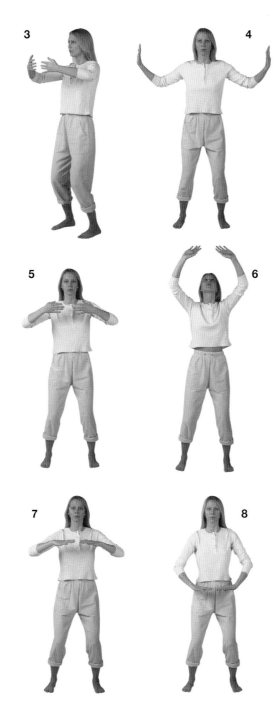

Alexander technique

Better breathing is made easier by the Alexander technique, a system of body awareness that works to correct "patterns of misuse" in the body's balance and structure.

Poor posture is linked to many breathing disorders. For instance, asthmatics often round their back and shoulders and thrust their neck forwards. Over time, this builds up into a pattern of muscular tension which is difficult to correct.

Developed by F.M. Alexander in the early 20th century, the Alexander technique is a system of re-educating the body to bring it back into alignment. It concentrates in particular on the dynamic relationship between the head, neck and back which are usually out of alignment.

The Alexander technique focuses on teaching how to perform simple movements – such as walking and sitting – correctly. It can be especially helpful for breathing disorders caused or exacerbated by poor posture and even stress.

Walking should be consciously directed. As the head leads and the body is aligned, the legs follow. It is also important that your eyes remain alert to your surroundings, as too much focus within cuts you off from your environment. Be careful not to wear clothes that restrict movement.

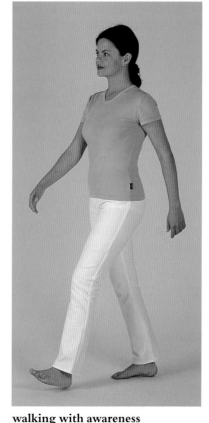

walking with awareness
To walk correctly, the head should lead the movement. The spine is straight, and the arms move freely at the sides.

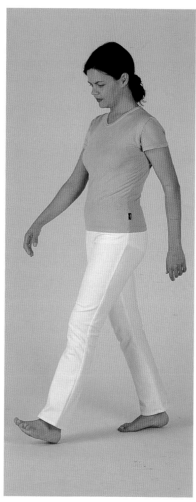

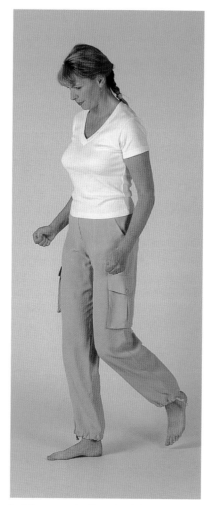

Here the the alignment between head, neck and back has been lost, allowing the head to drop at the neckline.

Correct alignment allows the whole body to lengthen and is especially important when moving up and down stairs. Leading with the head propels the body upwards and uses a minimum of energy when going up. When going down, the body moves in a free and more balanced way.

In this example, the shoulders are hunched and the arms are tense. The head is looking down when it should be held high and looking ahead.

Walking up stairs in this slumped position requires more effort to move both the body and legs. When descending stairs it is necessary to hold the legs in to avoid losing balance and so more energy is needed to support the system.

211

stretching with a partner

Gentle stretching exercises are a good way of opening the chest. Having a partner to help you stretch can be effective when you are suffering from mild breathing difficulties.

During episodes of mild asthma or bronchitis, working with a partner can feel very supportive. The following stretching exercises will ease muscular tension in the ribcage and encourage the chest to open.

stretching the lungs

This sequence of three stretches can help to counter the forward-bending hunched posture typical of someone with a shallow, rapid breathing pattern or congestive problems.

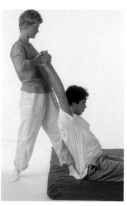

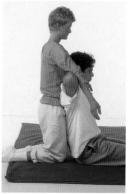

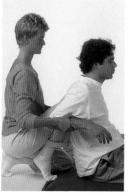

1 Sit your partner on the floor with legs straight. Stand behind, one foot in front of the other, and put the side of your leg against the spine. Take their hands, gripping the thumbs, and as you both exhale, lift up and lean back until your partner feels the stretch.

2 Kneel down behind your partner and ask them to clasp their hands behind their neck. Bring your arms in front of your partner's arms, and on the out-breath gently open up their elbows to the sides. Your partner should feel their chest opening.

3 Bring one knee up to support your partner's lower back and take hold of their lower arms. On the out-breath, bring their elbows towards each other, stretching to the middle of their back.

opening up the chest

This sequence of three exercises will improve lung energy, helping to promote relaxation and deeper breathing, which in turn regulates and enhances the flow of energy through the body. Try to breathe in through your nose and out through your mouth during the exercise.

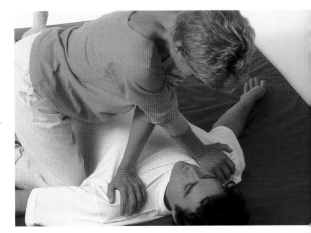

1 Cross your arms over and place the palms of your hands on your partner's shoulders. Ask your partner to breathe in and on the out-breath gradually bring your body weight over your hands, to stimulate the first point of the lung meridian (or energy channel) and gently open the chest. Repeat three times.

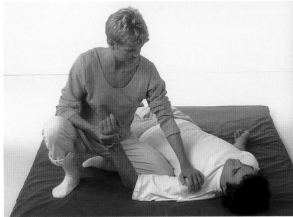

2 Keep your left hand on the shoulder and take a firm hold of your partner's left hand with your right hand. Lift the arm from the floor, shake it out and allow it to relax again.

3 Hold on to the thumb and give the left arm and the lung meridian an invigorating stretch.

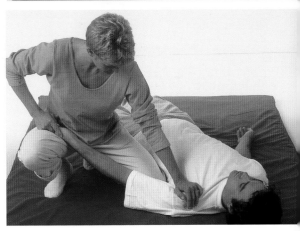

back & chest massage

The soothing pressure of a back and chest massage is an effective treatment for relaxing the diaphragm, easing congestion in the airways and encouraging the expulsion of excess mucus.

Excess mucus production is associated with many breathing disorders, from a viral infection such as a cold, to allergic symptoms associated with hay fever or the persistent "plugs" of mucus that block the airways in asthma and bronchitis.

simple three-step back massage

Make sure your partner is lying on a firm, but comfortable, surface and that the room is warm and draught-free. Keep their lower body covered with a towel or blanket as you work. You may like to use a little massage oil, such as sweet almond.

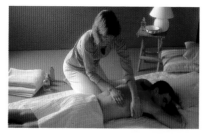

2 Move to your partner's side, and using the whole of your hand, pull the skin up very gently, one hand after the other, working all the way up and down one side of your partner's back a few times. Repeat on the other side.

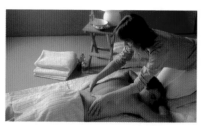

1 Position yourself at your partner's head and use a smooth stroking movement, down either side of the spine, with your thumbs. Take your hands to the side and glide back up to the shoulders.

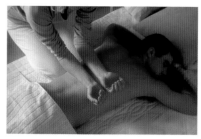

3 Stretch the back, by pressing your forearms and gliding them in opposite directions. As you work try to keep a steady pressure, lifting your arms when they reach the neck and buttocks. Return to the centre of the back and repeat twice more.

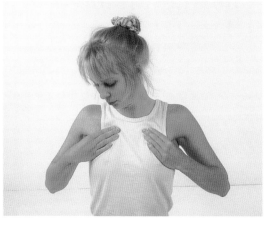

chest and abdomen releaser

A tight, tense chest will make congestion worse because trapped mucus is unable to move freely. Back and chest massage is a particularly effective cold treatment that also helps to boost immunity and eliminate toxins from the body.

1 Using the thumb and fingers, take a good grip of the pectoral muscles, leading from the chest towards the shoulder, and knead them firmly.

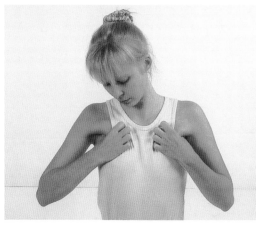

2 Be careful if you have any tenderness in the lymph glands under the armpits; women should also go gently if they have tender, swollen breasts, for example when pre-menstrual.

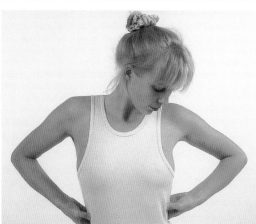

3 Using a couple of fingers feel in between the ribs for the intercostal muscles, and work firmly along between each rib moving the fingers in tiny circles, repeating on each side.

deepening the breath

If you are to practise active relaxation, you need to be aware of your breathing patterns. In yoga, the awareness of exhalation comes first, avoiding any forceful inhalation.

breath awareness

To do this exercise, sit upright on a sturdy chair, with your legs apart and feet planted firmly on the floor. Feel your breathing muscles working by placing your hands on your ribs, then your lower chest, then abdomen. The lower you can take the breathing movement, the more energized and relaxed you will feel. In yoga, you should always breathe out through the nose unless instructed otherwise.

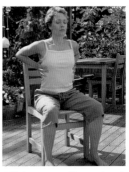

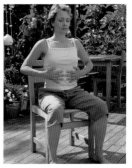

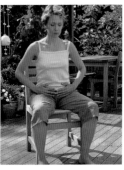

1 Bring your elbows back to open your chest, and place your hands on the sides of your ribs with fingers forward. Breathe in deeply, expanding your ribcage against your hands, then out, keeping the lift and openness in the chest. Be careful not to collapse, even though your ribcage contracts a little. Repeat.

2 Still with the elbows wide and chest open, bring the hands forward so that the little fingers rest against the lowest ribs. As you breathe in, you will feel the lower ribs expand outwards and the diaphragm contract downwards. As you exhale, you should feel the ribs relax inwards and your diaphragm upwards.

3 Now move your hands below the navel to feel the effect of deep breathing on the abdominals. Keep the shoulders relaxed. As you inhale, contracting the diaphragm, pressure flushes away stale blood from these organs. As you breathe out, pressure is released and fresh new blood rushes in, bringing oxygen and nutrients.

Breathing disorders are often associated with poor posture. Rolfing is a type of massage that aims to realign the body by working with its connective tissue.

Rolfing was developed by Dr Ida Rolf (1896–1979), an American biochemist. It aims to realign the body so that it can move in harmony with the forces of gravity. When the body structure is correctly balanced, we experience improved health and well-being.

Rolfing uses deep tissue massage to remould the body's connective tissue. While the technique can be rather painful at times, this is usually temporary and can be completely outweighed by the relief from chronic pain and discomfort caused by poor postural alignment. Although rolfing is not aimed at specific conditions, it has helped many asthma sufferers, as well as those suffering painful muscular conditions.

Rolfing often does more than simply remedy the body's structural problems, however. It is a holistic form of treatment that works on the whole person: body, mind and emotions. It recognizes that most physical problems also have a mental and emotional component. Problems with the lungs and respiration are often seen in people who have difficulties with letting go of painful experiences, especially those that happened a long time ago. When we are unable to process these experiences properly, it is as though they become "trapped" or stored in the body tissue and our system becomes clogged with "emotional junk". Consequently, during a rolfing treatment, manipulating deep-seated muscular tension can very often provoke an emotional release, such as crying or shouting.

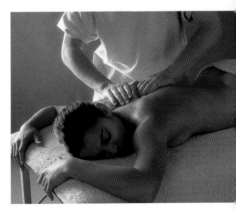

▸ *Rolfing is a form of deep tissue massage that helps to release tension and improve breathing patterns.*

osteopathy

Based on a series of manipulative techniques, osteopathy aims to realign the body's structure. It has been used to remedy many chronic respiratory conditions.

Osteopathy was founded by American doctor Andrew Still (1828–1917). It looks back to the fourth-century BC Hippocratic school of medical thought, in that it stresses the essential unity of all body parts and the body's innate self-healing mechanism.

Still identified the musculoskeletal system as a key element of health. Although we stand upright, our anatomy is still basically that of a creature which moves on all fours, and there is a constant strain on the whole framework. He recognized that the effect of gravity is particularly severe on the spine and that misalignment of the body's structure compromises health.

Osteopathy uses manipulative techniques that treat the whole body. These range from gentle, repeated movements of the joints to increase their mobility, to quick thrusting movements that rapidly guide the joint through its normal range. These latter manipulations often cause the clicking noise that many people experience during a session. An osteopathic treatment may also be accompanied by deep tissue massage.

Osteopathy works on the body's structure, so it can help redress postural problems linked to chronic breathing problems. These include a rounded back and shoulders and "collapsed" chest, as well as tightness around the intercostal muscles. It can also help with the back pain that many chronic asthma and bronchitis sufferers experience as a secondary symptom of their condition.

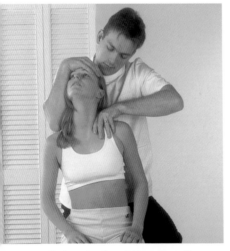

▲ During a treatment, the osteopath uses a series of manipulations to realign the body. This can help ease breathing problems.

216 reflexology for respiratory relief

Also known as "zone therapy", reflexology can be helpful for a range of respiratory conditions. It works by stimulating specific pressure points on the feet or hands.

Reflexology is based on the idea that areas on the feet are linked along invisible nerve channels or energy pathways to different organs and systems of the rest of the body. By working on the appropriate area of the feet, it is possible to affect the respiratory system.

the chest reflex points

The ball of each foot represents either side of the chest and is where the reflex points to the respiratory system are found. The whole area is bounded by the diaphragm, the reflex that lies across the base of the ball of each foot.

breathing relief

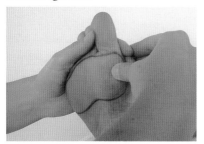

1 Using a firm thumb pressure, work the whole chest area to relieve congestion in the chest and lungs.

2 Fingerwalk the same area on the top of the feet to stimulate the chest lymph; this should encourage the removal of toxins.

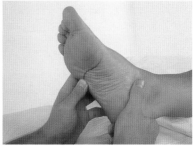

3 To relax the diaphragm, use a pressing movement with your thumb along the diaphragm line (the boundary where the ball of the foot meets the instep).

acupressure

By applying pressure to certain points on the body, it is possible to ease congestion in the lungs and sinuses, open up the airways and reduce symptoms of stress and tension.

Acupressure, which is based on very similar principles to shiatsu, uses finger pressure to stimulate and rebalance the energy flow along these meridians. It can be a useful quick-fix treatment that you can do on yourself (or with a partner) whenever you have a spare moment.

anxiety calmer

Rapid, shallow breathing or a tense "held-in" breath are often connected with anxiety and panic. In acupressure, there is a point known as the "Palace of Anxiety" that is located

near the base of the thumb. Pressing into this point will have a calming and relaxing effect and should help your breathing to slow down and deepen.

self-treatment for sinus relief

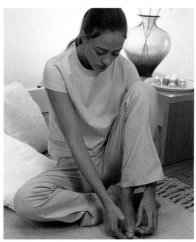

To relieve sinus congestion it can be helpful to work on foot acupressure points. Squeeze and press the tips of your toes and press and slide down their sides to the pads beneath. Continue this pressure, particularly on the big toes. To relieve a frontal sinus headache, apply pressure to just below the nail of the big toe.

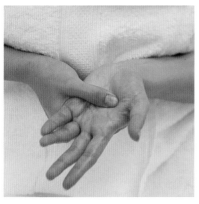

▲ Pressing into the pressure point near the base of the thumb can release tension.

Bring the scent of forest pine into your home – add a few drops of the essential oil to a vaporizer and enjoy a quick-fix treatment to unblock a stuffy nose.

219 aromatic compress

Essential oils can have a dramatic influence on the respiratory system. A compress is a good way to use them without the risk of irritating the delicate mucous membranes.

Inhalation is one of the fastest ways of using essential oils, but it is not always well tolerated, especially when the nasal passages and bronchi are inflamed and irritated. There are many essential oils that can help with hay fever, rhinitis and allergic asthma. Some of the most gentle, but still effective, include camomile and lemon balm (melissa), both of which are natural antihistamines and useful for treating allergy-related breathing problems. Camomile has a calming, anti-inflammatory effect and is especially useful for over-sensitivity. Lemon balm, too, can calm the antispasmodic "reflex reaction" that happens in allergic conditions.

compresses

A cool compress is best for inflamed conditions. To make one, you need a piece of soft, clean cotton and a small bowl of water. Add 4–6 drops of oil to the water and stir to disperse the oils. Soak the cloth in the water, squeeze it lightly and place over the upper back or chest. Leave it in position for about 30–45 minutes, making sure you stay warm and comfortable.

> **YEAR-ROUND ALLERGIES**
> Allergic rhinitis is an allergic condition that persists throughout the year with the same sort of symptoms as hay fever – watery eyes, sneezing and a runny nose. It can be caused by a variety of triggers, the most common ones being house dust, pet fur, artificial perfumes and chemicals.

▲ *A cool, aromatic compress will soothe inflamed and painful sinuses.*

steam inhalation

A steam inhalation is one of the most beneficial treatments for clearing the airways of congestion and encouraging better breathing. Adding certain essential oils can make it even more effective.

Rose oil helps to promote a feeling of general well-being but it is also helpful for treating respiratory and circulatory ailments such as palpitations, coughs and allergies affecting the lungs. To make it, the fresh petals of the flower have to be harvested early in the morning and then distilled immediately in order to capture as much of the essence as possible before it dissipates.

There are several varieties of chamomile, but Roman chamomile and German chamomile are the two most commonly used. The former is a creeping perennial with tiny needle-like leave; the latter is a taller upright annual with feathery leaves. Both bear a mass of white, daisy-like flowers. Chamomile is relaxing and anti-spasmodic, which is why it helps to relieve dry, tickly coughs.

steamy aroma

Inhalation is the quickest way for essential oil molecules to be absorbed into the body. To make a steam inhalation, fill a basin with 600ml/ 1 pint/2½ cups of boiling water and add 3 drops of rose essential oil and 4 drops of chamomile essential oil. Sit over the bowl making a "tent" with a towel around your head and inhale the vapours. If you experience any discomfort, stop immediately – sometimes, asthmatics cannot tolerate this form of treatment as it can feel claustrophobic and induce feelings of anxiety and panic.

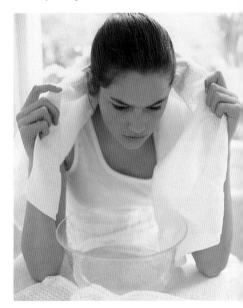

▲ *An oil-enriched steam inhalation can help ease congestion.*

221 soothing chest rub

A chest rub is an old-fashioned remedy for helping to clear congestion from the lungs. It is easy to make your own aromatic rub, using a base cream and essential oils.

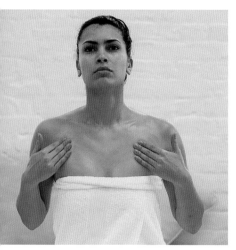

▲ *Using a gentle but firm pressure, rub a little aromatic cream into your upper chest. The essential oils, combined with a soothing massage, will have a therapeutic effect.*

For thick, chesty coughs and bronchitis, some of the most useful oils are frankincense, myrrh and benzoin. All have a calming, expectorant action on the body.

Frankincense is one of the most useful essential oils for the respiratory system; it slows and deepens the breathing and also has a calming, comforting effect. Both myrrh and benzoin (resinoid) have especially strong expectorant properties. Benzoin has a rich, vanilla-like aroma and is one of the main ingredients in "Friar's Balsam" cough mixture, a traditional syrup for easing chesty coughs. Myrrh also has a balsamic, slightly musty aroma and is especially helpful for clearing excess mucus. It has a slightly sedating effect and is good to use last thing at night.

All these oils are resinous and thus quite "heavy" fragrances, so you may prefer to use one or two of them as a base and combine with light-smelling oils such as lavender, herbaceous scents such as thyme or camphorous aromas such as eucalyptus, all of which have an affinity with the respiratory system.

aromatic cream recipe
To make a chest rub, add 5 drops of essential oil to a 50ml jar of unscented base cream. Blend the oil(s) into the cream using a cocktail stick (toothpick) or teaspoon handle. Rub the cream in well before going to bed, using a soothing circular stroke. The cream will keep for 2–3 months.

222 lavender sinus massage

Lavender is probably the most versatile essential oil. It has a gentle, balancing action on the body and a refreshing, distinctive scent. Use it to clear blocked and painful sinuses.

Inflammation of the sinus area around the nose and/or eyes causes chronic congestion, catarrh, headaches and breathing difficulties. It is a painful condition that is exacerbated by allergic reactions or colds. Lavender is a natural analgesic (painkiller) and also has antiseptic and antibiotic properties. Its healing, soothing qualities make it ideal for treating painful sinus problems.

quick-fix self-massage sequence
To make a massage oil mixture, add 4–5 drops lavender essential oil to 30ml (2 tbsp) sweet almond oil, and stir to blend. As you massage your face, take great care to ensure that you keep the oil well away from your eyes.

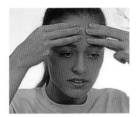

1 Place your hands just above the mid-point between the eyebrows. Make small circles with your fingers, working your way across the forehead. Apply gentle pressure.

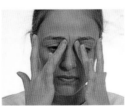

2 Place your middle fingers at either side of your nose. Breathe in, and on the out-breath press firmly for a few seconds, then release. Repeat three times.

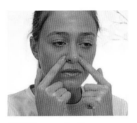

3 With your index fingers on either side of your nose, press gently, holding and releasing. Repeat three times. This is an important pressure point for opening up the sinuses.

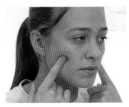

4 Draw your fingers along the cheekbones applying pressure strokes. Then use your thumbs to make small circular movements along this line.

223 healing bath oils

Essential oils in the bath have a two-fold effect: they are absorbed through the skin while their aroma is inhaled, having an immediate effect on the respiratory system.

Sandalwood is widely used in Ayurvedic medicine, the ancient healing system of India, where it has many medicinal uses, especially in the treatment of bacterial infections. In the West, aromatherapists use sandalwood to treat many different conditions, including chronic bronchitis and respiratory disorders that are characterized by a dry, irritating and tickly cough. Some

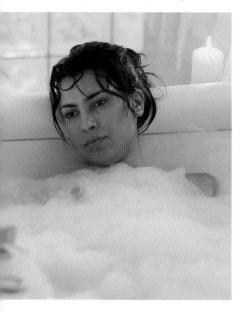

people prefer the scent of sandalwood to the more floral fragrances. Alternatively, marjoram is effective for respiratory conditions. According to Culpeper, the 17th-century English herbalist, it "helpeth all diseases of the chest which hinder the freeness of breathing". It seems particularly effective with asthma, bronchitis and colds, and for relaxing spasmodic, tickly coughs. It can also loosen mucus and, if used at the early onset of a cold, may prevent it turning into a nasty chest infection that is much harder to shift.

essential oil bathing
Both marjoram and sandalwood have a sedative effect, and are thus good choices to use in a bedtime bath. To use essential oils in the bath, run the water first and then add 4–5 drops of oil. Swirl the water to disperse the oils. For maximum benefit, soak in the water for at least ten minutes.

◄ *An aromatic sandalwood bath can ease a dry cough and promote a good night's sleep. Breathe deeply as you soak to experience the full healing effect of the essential oil.*

224 homeopathy for better breathing

Based on a "like cures like" principle, homeopathy stimulates the body's naturally well-balanced self-healing mechanism. Homeopathy offers a range of remedies to help breathing disorders.

Conventional science has as yet no plausible explanation for homeopathic medicine. The remedies are prepared from plant, animal and mineral substances that are diluted to such an extent that no molecules of the original substance remain. Practitioners claim, however, that homeopathy is a form of vibrational or energy medicine: that what remains in the remedy is the "energetic blueprint" of the original substance, which works on the body's subtle energy system, rather than directly on the physical body.

A homeopathic remedy is selected by matching it to your particular physical, mental and emotional symptoms. This list will help you match a remedy to your symptoms. Take a 6c potency pill, three times a day, until your symptoms improve.

first–aid for hay fever and rhinitis
ALLIUM CEPA: burning nasal discharge and watery eyes.
ARSENICUM: burning eyes with tears that feel hot; sneezing brings no relief.
EUPHRASIA: profuse runny nose which blocks at night; eyes feel sore.

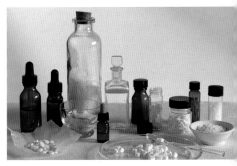

▲ Homeopathic remedies are highly diluted. They are available in pill and tincture form.

first–aid for sinusitis
HEPAR SULPH: painful swelling of the nasal cavities with yellow mucus.
NAT MUR: profuse watery discharge; sneezing, frontal headache.
SILICA: dry blocked nose, severe headache with bouts of sneezing; worse for cold, better for warmth.

first–aid for coughs
BRYONIA: dry, hacking cough, made worse by changes in temperature.
IPECAC: spasmodic cough with rattly mucus on the chest.
PHOSPHORUS: hoarse voice, dry tickly cough and a tight feeling like a band around the chest.

225 reiki for the chest & lungs

Originating in Japan, reiki is a form of spiritual healing that is very gentle and non-invasive. It is particularly useful for breathing problems associated with panic and anxiety.

In Japanese, "rei-ki" can be translated as "universal-life energy". A treatment involves channelling this cosmic energy, or light, to where it is most needed in the body. To give a treatment, visualize a stream of golden light entering the crown of your head, pouring through your body and constantly flowing out through your hands as you work.

treating the upper chest
When we work on the upper chest area we are also connecting with the energies of the heart. A shallow breathing pattern and tension in the upper chest may be associated with emotional hurts and disappointments that have become "locked" in the body. Channelling reiki to this area can help to release these in a way that is comforting and soothing.

The hand position shown here works for many people who visibly relax, absorbing the reiki into the lymph region. This is a great help in ridding the body of toxins. The position also treats the lungs and clears the chest, making it effective for asthma sufferers and smokers.

releasing tension in the chest

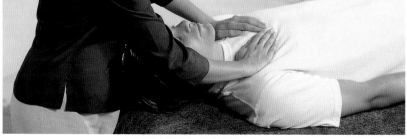

Sitting or standing at your partner's head, place your hands in an inverted "V" position at the top of the chest. Holding this position soothes and relaxes tension and is also a tonic for the lungs. Do not place pressure on your partner; if necessary rest your elbows on the treatment couch so that you are steady.

colour therapy

Bringing colour energies into the body is another way of rebalancing body and soul. It is particularly useful for breathing problems with a strong emotional component.

Colour is light vibrating at a particular frequency, with colours at the red end of the spectrum having a lower frequency than those at the blue end. Each band of colour has different qualities and associations that can be used for healing. This visualization is a simple but effective way of bringing the healing power of colour into your body – it can also indicate which colour energies you are most in need of absorbing.

BETTER BREATHING WITH COLOUR
red: "emotional" asthma characterized by insecurity and nervousness.
orange: clears mucus; therapeutic for hay fever.
yellow: strengthens resistance to allergic reactions and colds.
green: expansive; relaxes tense chest muscles; useful for asthma and other respiratory problems.
blue and indigo: calms over-excited or agitated states; useful for desensitizing allergic reactions.
violet: speeds up the body's healing processes; balancing.

rainbow breathing

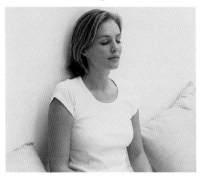

1 Sit with eyes closed in a comfortable position. Relax and allow your breathing to slow and settle.

2 Imagine the air around you is a rich, deep red. As you breathe in, imagine that your whole body fills with red energy. Continue breathing in the red light, then imagine breathing it out through your feet into the earth.

3 Repeat step two, this time imagining the air is a vibrant, warm orange colour. When you have finished with orange, continue with the other colours of the rainbow: yellow, green, blue, indigo and violet.

chakra balancing

Disturbances in breathing are linked to imbalances in the chakra system. Working on the chakras of the upper body can help restore healthy breathing.

The chakras are subtle energy centres that run up the front and back of the body. Each chakra corresponds to different organs of the body and has colour and gemstone associations.

chakras of the upper body

The heart chakra is located at the centre of the chest and is related to the heart, lungs and arms. Its colour correspondence is green and its gemstone is rose quartz. The ears, nose and mouth are under the influence of the throat chakra, which also deals with communication and creative self-expression. Its colour is blue and its stone is turquoise. The brow chakra or "third eye" is in the centre of the forehead and relates to the pineal gland, which influences our mood and behaviour. Its colour is indigo and the gemstone is lapis lazuli.

rebalancing the chakras

For asthma and chronic chest complaints, concentrate on the heart chakra. For colds, hay fever and allergic rhinitis, focus on the throat chakra; and for sinus problems, work on the third eye.

Sit in a comfortable position with your eyes closed. Place your hands over the corresponding chakra. Take a deep breath into the area and hold the breath for as long as feels comfortable; then breathe out. If you want to use gemstones and/or colour, either visualize the colour or hold the appropriate stone, or a crystal, over the chakra as you breathe.

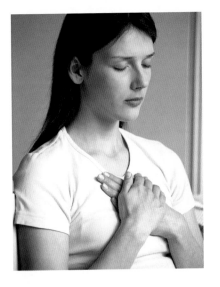

◄ *Focusing on the heart chakra can have a soothing effect on the respiratory system.*

228

flower essences

Some breathing disorders have a strong mental and emotional component. Flower essences are useful for treating negative emotional states and restoring balance.

Bach flower essences can be useful for breathing problems that have a strong emotional component or are made worse by stress, such as asthma or hyperventilation (panic attacks). Select a remedy by matching your symptoms to the remedy description. A good way to start is to make a list of the three to five main issues that are troubling you. If you find making a selection difficult, consult an experienced practitioner who will be able to guide you towards making the right decision.

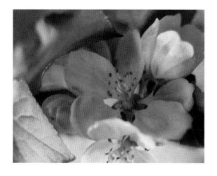

▲ The cleansing action of crab apple can help clear mucus from the airways.

Bach flower remedy selector

ASPEN: fearful of the dark, of dying, of the future.

CRAB APPLE: cleanser and detoxifier.

IMPATIENS: tense and irritable, often with a headache.

MIMULUS: anxious and fearful for known causes.

WHITE CHESTNUT: a mind that will not switch off.

OLIVE: mentally and physically drained and exhausted.

ROCK ROSE: severe panic; terror, fright, hysteria.

RESCUE REMEDY: multi–purpose first–aid remedy for shock and panic.

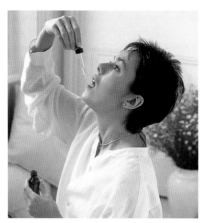

▲ Flower essences may be taken in water or undiluted. Take 2–3 drops.

229 fortifying garlic

Since ancient times, garlic has been valued as a powerful herbal medicine for strengthening the respiratory system and building immunity. It is an effective preventative measure.

Garlic was widely used to treat all kinds of infection before antibiotics were developed. It can be strengthening and revitalizing, and, because its volatile oil is largely excreted through the lungs, it has an affinity with the respiratory system.

Ideally, garlic is best eaten raw, but if you dislike its pungent taste and odour, try it lightly stir-fried, making sure it does not go brown and bitter. Alternatively, take 1–3 garlic capsules daily as a preventative measure.

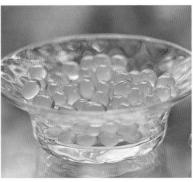

▲ A convenient way of taking garlic is as odourless capsules or pearls. Take 1–3 a day.

walnut and garlic sauce

This flavoursome sauce comes from the Mediterranean regions, and is delicious served with roast chicken or steamed vegetables.

2 slices white bread, crusts removed
60ml/4 tbsp milk
150g/5oz/1¼ cups shelled walnuts
4 garlic cloves, chopped
120ml/4fl oz/½ cup olive oil
15–30ml/1–2 tbsp walnut oil, plus extra oil for drizzling
juice of 1 lemon
salt and freshly ground black pepper
paprika, for dusting

Place the trimmed bread in a shallow dish, pour over the milk and leave it to soak for about five minutes. Transfer the bread mixture to a food processor or blender, and add the walnuts and chopped garlic, processing to a coarse paste. Gradually add the olive oil and walnut oil through a feeder tube to make a smooth, thick sauce. Stir in lemon juice to taste and season with salt and pepper. When ready to use, transfer the sauce to a small serving bowl, drizzle with a little extra walnut oil and dust the surface lightly with paprika.

230 protective echinacea

Purple coneflower, or echinacea, is one of the most powerful medicines in the Native American tradition. The plant has many healing properties and a strong affinity with the respiratory system.

Inspired by the plant's spiky central cone, the name echinacea is derived from the Greek *echinos*, meaning hedgehog. Echinacea can help the body fight off infections by boosting the immune system. While Native Americans have used echinacea to treat all kinds of illnesses, including poisonous bites, wounds and fevers, research has shown that it is also helpful for chronic infections, problems related to the upper respiratory tract, and allergies.

As a herbal remedy, echinacea is available in tincture or capsule form in good health stores and pharmacies.

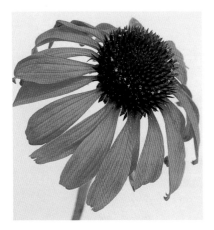

To treat colds and upper respiratory tract infections, take 2.5ml/½ tsp tincture diluted in water, or a 500mg capsule, three times a day. As a preventative measure, to strengthen the immune system, take 2.5ml/½ tsp tincture or a 500mg capsule once a day. Echinacea should not be taken for more than two or three weeks at a time, and should be avoided when pregnant or breastfeeding.

As well as boosting the immune system, echinacea can act as a tonic to balance it. Allergic conditions – such as hay fever, rhinitis and allergic asthma – are triggered when the immune system overreacts to a stimulant, such as pollen, dust or fur, or certain foods and chemicals. Not realizing these substances are harmless, the body mounts a full-scale defence against them, producing symptoms such as wheezing, sneezing, congestion, watery eyes, a runny nose. Echinacea can help to suppress this reaction and stabilize the immune system.

◀ *For colds, flu, bronchitis and other types of infection, echinacea gives the immune system a tremendous boost.*

231 healing herb tincture

The antiseptic and tonic action of thyme makes it a useful immunity-booster as well as an effective remedy for chest infections, such as pleurisy, bronchitis and whooping cough.

Culpeper, the 17th-century English herbalist, described thyme as a strengthener of the lungs and one of the best remedies for whooping cough. Thyme is a powerful expectorant and useful for treating viral chest infections.

Many herbs contain active ingredients that are not easily extracted by water or are destroyed by heat. A tincture solves these problems as well as preserving the extract. A tincture is an extract of a herb in a mixture of alcohol and water, normally 25 per cent alcohol strength, with the alcohol preserving the medicine for two years or more. As tinctures are concentrated extracts, they should only be used for short periods of time. Take 5ml/1tsp of tincture three times a day, diluted in water or fresh juice.

preparing a thyme tincture

200g/7oz dried or 300g/11oz
   fresh thyme
750ml/1¼ pints/3 cups water
250ml/8fl oz/1 cup vodka

Chop up the herb and place in a large glass storage jar. Pour on the alcohol and water, seal the jar and leave in a cool place for two weeks. Shake the jar occasionally. Pour the mixture through a piece of muslin (cheesecloth) into a clean jar or bottle, seal well and store in a cool place.

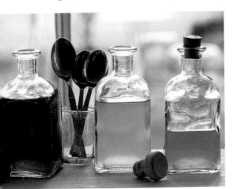

▲ Tinctures are concentrated medicinal extracts and should be used sparingly.

> **CAT'S THYME**
> A herb known as cat's thyme or *Marum verum* has been used as a form of snuff. It is said to reduce inflammation of the nasal passages and is a useful remedy for nasal polyps and snoring.

232 nettle & elderflower tisane

A tisane is a good way to use the more delicate parts of plants, especially their leaves and flowers. Try a combination of nettles and elderflower for a range of breathing disorders.

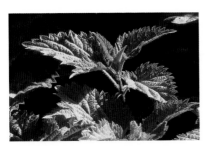

▲ Fresh nettle tops can be cooked and eaten as a vegetable or made into a tisane.

The warming action of nettles makes them useful for colds, while their anti-inflammatory and anti-allergic properties make them especially useful for asthma and hay fever. As well as being made into a drink, nettle leaves can also be lightly cooked and eaten as a vegetable. Eating cooked nettle tops in the springtime is said to be an effective detoxifier, helping to rid the body of excess phlegm accumulated during the winter.

Elderflowers can also be helpful for respiratory problems, including asthma and colds. Elderflower remedies have a relaxing and decongesting effect on the bronchi, thereby reducing muscle spasm and helping to expel excess mucus. They also have a toning effect on the mucous linings of the nose and throat and increase resistance to infection.

tisane recipe

Taken regularly for a few months before the hay fever season, a nettle and elderflower tisane can really help. It can also help to reduce catarrh, so is useful for colds, bronchitis and asthma. To make a tisane, pour a cup of near-boiling water on 5ml/1 tsp each of fresh chopped leaves and blossoms, or 2.5ml/½ tsp each of the dried herbs. Leave for 10–15 minutes. Strain and drink three times a day.

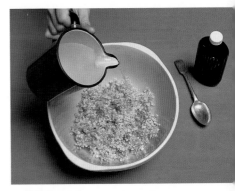

▲ Elderflower tisane can be made very simply from fresh blossoms and hot water.

233 easy-breathing tea

Herbal teas are an easy and convenient way of using herbal medicines. Some of the best herbal treatments for chest and sinus problems are yarrow, elderflowers, peppermint and elecampane.

One of nature's best "lung herbs" is elecampane, which is particularly useful for treating chronic bronchitis and bronchial asthma. Elecampane has a powerful anti-inflammatory and soothing action. It also reduces mucus secretions, is a powerful expectorant and stimulates the whole of the immune system.

Another plant known for its anti-inflammatory qualities is yarrow, it also has antiseptic, antispasmodic and anti-allergic properties, which make it useful for treating hay fever. It also acts as a tonic to the nervous system, and can help calm the irritated, anxious states associated with some breathing problems.

Elderflowers can be used to soothe an irritated respiratory system, while peppermint has invigorating antiseptic properties and is useful for clearing blocked sinuses and treating chesty colds. The antispasmodic action of peppermint makes it useful for easing bronchial spasm in asthma and for calming tension and anxiety; it is also a good warming herb for relieving winter colds and chills.

easy-breathing recipe

This recipe uses a combination of yarrow, peppermint, elecampane and elderflower in a tea that encourages the airways to open while protecting and invigorating the immune system. To make the tea you will need 2.5ml/ ½ tsp of each herb per 250ml/8fl oz/ 1 cup of near-boiling water. For fresh flowers and leaves, double the quantity of each herb. Add the herbs to the hot water and leave to steep for 5–10 minutes. Strain off the liquid and drink two or three times a day. Sweeten with honey to taste.

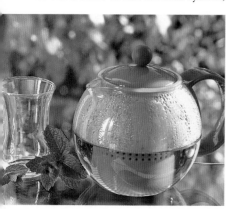

▲ It is easy to make your own herbal teas. Simply add the herb to hot water and infuse.

234 chamomile & eyebright infusion

In cases of hay fever and allergic rhinitis, chamomile and eyebright will treat physical and mental symptoms. The plants may be used separately or together in an infusion.

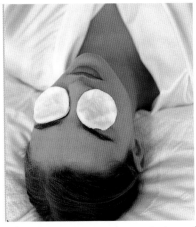

◀ To relieve the itchy, sore red eyes associated with hay fever, soak cotton pads in a chamomile and eyebright infusion.

There are two main varieties of chamomile, Roman and German, with similar properties, but it is German chamomile (*Matricaria recutica*) that is especially useful for hay fever and allergic asthma. This is due to some of its key constituents, which have a strong antispasmodic action, relieving irritability and promoting calm. Research has shown that chamomile is also a natural antihistamine, giving it an anti-allergic effect.

As its name suggests, eyebright (or euphrasia as it is sometimes known) can be helpful for treating allergic conditions such as hay fever and rhinitis that involve itchy, red and watery eyes. Eyebright has a tightening effect on the mucous membranes of the eyes and reduces inflammation. It also counters catarrh, making it useful for clearing the sinuses and the nasal passages. However, it is not recommended for a stuffy, blocked-up nose, but only for conditions where mucus is watery, profuse and free-flowing.

making an infusion

To make an infusion, pour a cup of near-boiling water on the herbs – using 5ml/1 tsp of each fresh chopped herb, or 2.5ml/½ tsp of dried herb. Leave to stand for 10–15 minutes, strain and use as required.

A chamomile and eyebright infusion can be used in two ways: first, as a tea to be taken two or three times a day; and secondly, by soaking pads of cotton wool in a cooled infusion and placing them on the eyelids to soothe sore, irritated eyes.

235 vitamin A

One of the most important vitamins for helping to maintain a healthy respiratory system is vitamin A. It guards against infection and helps protect the lungs against pollution.

Vitamin A can be stored by the body and need not be replenished every day. It occurs in two forms: first as preformed vitamin A, or retinol, and second as provitamin A, or carotene. The former is found only in foods of animal origin, while the second is provided by both plant and animal-derived foods.

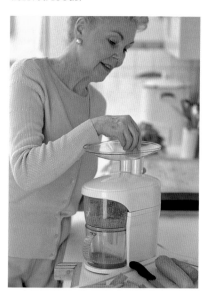

▲ *Carrots provide a versatile source of vitamin A. For maximum benefit, enjoy them raw, in salads or as a fresh juice.*

Some of the best natural sources of vitamin A are carrots, fish liver oil, liver, green and yellow vegetables, eggs, milk and dairy products. If you eat plenty of these foods you will provide your body with adequate vitamin A. However, some breathing problems are exacerbated by eating too many dairy products and eggs. It is also worth bearing in mind that foods lose their vitamins once they have been picked and stored, and that non-organic varieties may also contain traces of pesticides or antibiotics.

If you suffer from a serious respiratory condition, such as asthma, bronchitis, pleurisy or emphysema, you would probably do well to take a vitamin A supplement, at least until the symptoms improve. Supplements are usually available in two forms, one that is derived from fish oils – such as cod-liver oil – and another that is water-dispersible and recommended for anyone who has trouble tolerating oil, such as those suffering from oily skin, for example. A typical daily dose is 10,000 IU, but always check the label on the container to find out how many capsules to take.

236 vitamin B5

The B vitamins play an essential role in more than 60 metabolic reactions. B vitamins, particularly B5, are helpful for stress-related breathing problems, such as asthma and hyperventilation.

Also known as the anti-stress vitamin, B5 (or pantothenic acid) has been found to be particularly useful for treating stress. It is essential for every cell in the body and a deficiency leads to continuous colds and respiratory problems. Foods that contain high amounts of B5 are wholegrains, dried beans, eggs and nuts.

Of all the B vitamins, B6 (or pyridoxine) is probably the most important. It is involved in more bodily functions than almost any other nutrient and affects both physical and mental health. It is an immunity booster and has an affinity with the nervous system, making it helpful for treating allergies and asthma. However, the B vitamins generally work best when taken as a complex, as their effect is synergistic: in other words, the action of one enhances that of another.

Foods that are good natural sources of B vitamins include wheat germ, brewer's yeast, brown rice, fish, liver, eggs, milk and cheese as well as cabbage and avocados.

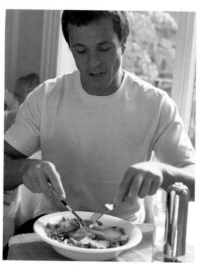

▲ Avocados provide plenty of B vitamins – add them to salads and sandwiches.

If your breathing problems are stress-related, it may help to take a B vitamin complex supplement, as B vitamins are used up more quickly when you are stressed. Look for a "time release" supplement, which means that the vitamins are contained in a special formula that will slowly release the nutrients over a seven- to eight-hour time period. A high-potency dose would be around 350mg a day.

Increase your intake of

vitamin C and eat

plenty of fresh fruit.

Vitamin C is a natural

antihistamine and will help

to keep hay fever and

allergies under control.

238 quercetin

A compound that is found in apples, tea, onions and red wine, quercetin is said to be helpful for allergy-related problems such as allergic rhinitis, asthma and hay fever.

Quercetin is a member of a large group of water-soluble plant compounds called flavonoids. It acts as an antihistamine, so it is helpful for calming allergic reactions, and it also has useful anti-inflammatory and antioxidant properties.

Quercetin may help to alleviate the symptoms of asthma, allergies and hay fever in some sufferers. Good natural sources include apples, raspberries, red grapes, citrus fruits, onions and leafy green vegetables. Alternatively, red wine and black and green tea also contain this flavonoid. Quercetin is also available as a supplement, available in good health stores and pharmacies: the recommended dose is 400mg two or three times a day.

WHAT ARE ALLERGIES?

An allergic reaction is a response mounted by the immune system to a certain food, inhalant (airborne substance), or chemical. Special immune cells called "mast cells" release histamine and other chemicals in order to destroy what the body perceives as a harmful substance. These chemicals cause inflammation and an increase in lymph fluid, and act as a signal for more mast cells to join in.

A typical allergic attack starts with itching in the nose and eyes, followed by watering of the eyes and nose as the body tries to flush out its invaders. Sneezing often comes next – an attempt to remove them more forcibly.

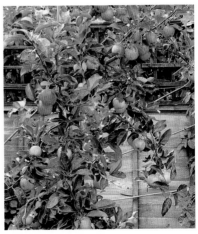

▲ Studies have linked eating five or more apples (rich in quercetin) a week with improved lung function and a lower risk of respiratory diseases such as asthma, bronchitis and emphysema.

239 zinc-fuelled foods

A powerful immunity-booster, zinc is an essential mineral that is required for more than 200 enzyme activities within the body. It can help protect against colds and allergies.

Zinc protects the immune system, and is vital for normal cell division and function, yet many of us are zinc-deficient. Frequent colds, a poor sense of taste or smell and feeling run-down are signs of a deficiency. Stress, sweating – through vigorous exercise for instance – smoking and high tea, coffee, alcohol and refined food consumption all deplete zinc reserves.

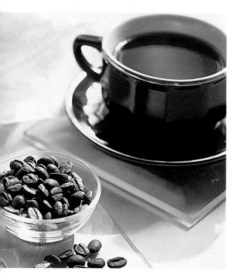

▲ *Coffee may have a tempting aroma, but it is worth remembering that it depletes your body's zinc reserves.*

Asthmatics and those suffering from chronic chest problems are particularly vulnerable to colds and flu. To strengthen your immunity, consider taking a zinc supplement of 15–20mg a day with a glass of orange juice (vitamin C aids zinc absorption). Zinc supplements should not be taken on an empty stomach because they may make you feel sick. Zinc lozenges are also available for colds and sore throats: it seems that zinc may have a direct effect on the cold viruses in the mouth, nose and throat and stop them from multiplying.

zinc-fuelled soft-shelled crab
Coat the crabs lightly in flour seasoned with pepper and fry in 60ml/4 tbsp very hot oil until they are golden brown, 2–3 minutes each side. Drain them on kitchen paper and keep hot. Gently cook 2 sliced chillies and 4 chopped spring onions in the oil for 2 minutes. Sprinkle with a generous pinch of salt then spread over the crabs. Serve two small crabs per person on a bed of shredded lettuce, mooli (daikon) and carrot with light soy sauce for dipping.

240

say "no" to...

What we eat has a direct bearing on our health and fitness. Certain foods are known to aggravate breathing problems so it may help to avoid them and look for healthier options.

The number of people suffering from asthma and allergies has risen dramatically in the last 50 years. During this time our diet has changed quite radically, and our consumption of refined and highly processed foods, that are far from their natural state, has increased dramatically.

what to avoid

Research has shown that refined carbohydrates depress the immune system within one hour of being consumed. These include all products containing white flour or sugar – bread, biscuits, cake and pasta, as well as sweets and chocolate. For a tasty snack, eat fresh fruit, nuts or cereal bars instead. It may also be that a diet high in animal fats reduces the immune system's efficiency, while sugar and wheat are another two foodstuffs that weaken immunity, and also contribute to the formation of mucus. Honey is a natural alternative to sugar, and if you want to avoid wheat, you can try eating more of other grains such as millet, rye, or rice. Rice cakes make a low-calorie, healthy alternative to bread.

Milk, eggs and cheese are a good source of calcium but may encourage mucus production. Try substituting calcium-enriched soya milk instead of cow's milk, or you may find your body tolerates goat's or sheep's milk better.

Finally, foods that contain artificial colourings, flavourings and preservatives can aggravate asthma and allergies and are best avoided.

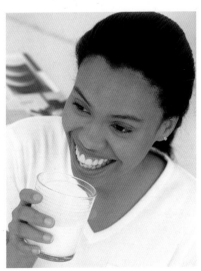

▲ Calcium-enriched soya milk is a good substitute for cow's milk as it helps to ensure you are getting the calcium you need.

241

say "yes" to...

The healing power of food was recognized by Hippocrates, the "father of medicine", more than 2,000 years ago. And there are certain foods that can help to support better breathing.

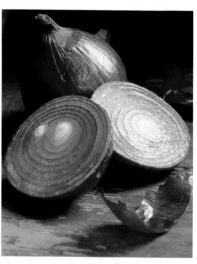

▲ Onions have a long tradition as a healing food for asthma and respiratory problems.

To keep your body healthy it is important to eat a varied and balanced diet, including as much fresh, organic produce as possible. Dark green vegetables such as broccoli, cabbage and spinach, as well as root vegetables such as carrots, turnips and onions, are all good for respiratory problems. Oily fish, such as salmon, mackerel and herring, help the immune system, while millet is a particularly low-allergenic food, and brown rice is known for its calming effect on the nervous system.

healing onions

As well as having cleansing and detoxifying properties, onions are a natural antibiotic and antiseptic and have an antispasmodic effect. It is for these reasons that onions are a traditional treatment for asthma, as they are believed to reduce bronchial spasm.

quick-fix onion soup

2 large onions
15ml/1 tbsp sunflower oil
1 litre/1¾ pints/4 cups stock (chicken or vegetable)
fresh thyme
½ tsp / 2.5ml yeast extract
black pepper

Peel and chop the onions. Heat the oil in a heavy pan and soften the onions, taking care not to brown them. Add the stock, thyme, yeast extract and pepper. Bring to the boil and simmer gently for 15–20 minutes. Pour the soup into bowls and serve.

check it out

Smoking aside, allergies and intolerances are probably the most common single cause of respiratory problems. Adverse food reactions are linked to many of these problems.

True food allergies are potentially life-threatening, but are relatively rare. Food intolerances, however, are more common, but they are often difficult to detect. Many people believe they are linked to allergies.

COMMON FOOD INTOLERANCES

cereals: wheat is the main problem, although rye is another culprit.

cow's milk: dairy products such as cheese and butter made from cow's milk.

shellfish: mussels, prawns, crab, lobster, scallops.

eggs: an egg allergy is often found in asthmatics.

yeast: found in bread, fermented products such as wine and beer, and yeast extract spreads.

nuts: especially walnuts and hazelnuts.

food additives: these include sulphites (preservatives found in many foods and difficult to isolate); tartrazine (a yellow colouring); MSG (monosodium glutamate, a flavour-enhancer that is widely used in Chinese cooking).

the elimination diet

The best way to check for a food intolerance is by eliminating suspect foods from your diet to see if your symptoms improve. This can be tricky as many common triggers are found in a huge variety of everyday foods, so you will need to check the labels of everything you buy. Cut out all the common triggers for a couple of weeks and keep to a fairly plain diet until your symptoms improve. You may then reintroduce the food groups, one by one; if your symptoms don't return after two or three days, that food or food group is probably safe for you.

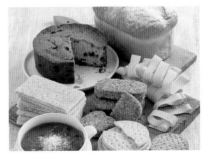

▲ A wheat intolerance is quite common. Wheat-containing foods include bread, cake, pasta, wheat, cereals, biscuits and processed soups.

body cleanse

When breathing problems are associated with thick catarrh that just won't seem to shift, then a detox or body cleanse may be what is required. A fresh juice fast is a good way to start.

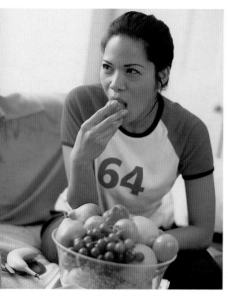

▲ *Detoxing with fresh fruit gives your digestive system a rest and can help clear mucus from the body.*

The bacteria that populate the colon and the small intestine have an important part to play in health, including the health of the respiratory system. In fact, it is estimated that 70 per cent of our lymphatic defence system, essential for fighting infection, lies in the bowel wall.

The delicate balance of our intestinal environment can be upset by many things, including stress, eating the wrong foods and taking synthetic drugs. Allergies and the over-production of mucus are signs that the body's internal balance is out of kilter. A body cleanse or detox can give your body a chance to rest and repair itself.

2-day detox plan
Based on fruit and vegetable dishes and juices, this gentle and effective detox is ideal for a quiet weekend.

• Morning: Kick-start your liver with a cup of hot water and lemon juice. For breakfast, prepare a fruit juice and dilute with water. Eat a small bunch of grapes or an apple mid-morning.
• Afternoon: Prepare a vegetable juice and a large salad for lunch, for example, tomatoes, cucumber, fennel, carrot and beetroot (beet). Drink plenty of water, either bottled mineral or filtered tap water.
• Evening: Eat a dinner consisting of very lightly steamed vegetables, sprinkled with fresh herbs and lemon juice, along with some brown rice.

Bake an apple with an orange and a lemon, both studded with cloves. Chop the fruits, add finely grated ginger and brown sugar. Steep in boiling water for an hour; strain into a pitcher when cool and pour in bitter lemon. This mulled drink will help you breathe.

At work we are subjected to a range of potential "allergens" that can be problematic for asthma and allergies. These include chemicals, dust and electromagnetic pollution.

A typical office contains a vast array of electronic equipment, including computers, laser printers, scanners and photocopiers, as well as telephones – both land lines and mobiles. Research shows that the electromagnetic radiation emitted by such equipment interferes with the body's electromagnetic field and may be linked to health problems and a general weakening of our immunity.

If you suffer breathing problems it is particularly important to protect yourself against these potentially harmful influences, as a weakened immune system increases the likelihood of your condition getting worse. Make sure you take regular breaks away from your computer and keep potted plants and quartz crystals near electronic equipment to help absorb the energy waves. Lack of natural light can also be a problem so make sure your work area uses bulbs that simulate natural daylight rather than fluorescent tube lighting.

toxic substances

There are also many environmental toxins. In an office, the laser carbon in photocopiers and printers can trigger an allergic reaction – sneezing, shortness of breath and watery eyes. Make sure you sit as far away from this equipment as possible, and if possible avoid changing the toner cartridge. Chemicals in paint, glue, cleaning products and even felt-tipped pens can also provoke a reaction, while various dusts (from wood or cotton for instance), fumes, gases and aerosol mists or sprays can be extremely damaging.

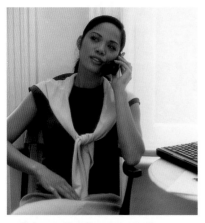

▲ *Being continually surrounded by electronic equipment can harm our body's systems.*

at home

Far from being a safe haven, the home can be one of the biggest culprits when it comes to provoking allergic reactions. However, there are steps you can take to make it an allergy-free zone.

Some of the most common environmental allergens around the home include house dust, pet fur and mould spores, although toxic chemicals used in cleaning materials, furniture, flooring and paint can also be involved.

dust mites

A typical mattress may contain as many as two million dust mites, but it is the droppings rather than the mites that are the problem. These are found in dust, so keep your home as dust-free as possible. Regular vacuuming and washing and airing of bedding can help; an anti-allergenic mattress and pillow covers are also a good idea.

Fitted carpets, central heating and double-glazing, while very comfortable and convenient, can make allergies worse – they provide a warm environment in which germs breed. If your allergies are worse during the night, then sleep with the window open if possible, even in the winter, and see if there is any improvement in your symptoms.

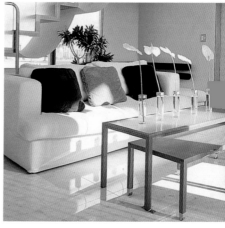

▲ If your home is free from clutter, it will be easier to keep clean and dust-free.

other allergens

Mould thrives in humid conditions, so keeping your home dry and well-aired is the best solution. Cats and other household pets are a common trigger of allergic reactions, in which case the only practical solution is to avoid them. Chemicals such as formaldehyde and wood preservatives are poisonous to allergic individuals; foam furniture, chipboard and wooden furniture and flooring may contain these substances.

outdoor hazards

There are many different kinds of airborne substances that can irritate the sensitive mucous membranes of the respiratory system, including a variety of pollens and man-made pollutants.

Air pollution has reached record levels. A range of poisonous gases, including ozone, sulphur dioxide and carbon monoxide, and "particulate matter", such as soot and dust, are released into the air by transport and industry. People with lung disease (such as asthma or emphysema) may be very sensitive to air pollution.

ozone levels

In cities, the worst offender is ground-level ozone, created when engine and fuel gases are affected by sunlight. This is why ozone levels increase on a bright, sunny day when the air is still. Recorded on the Air Quality Index, these levels are cited daily in the local media. If pollution aggravates your problems, then you should check this index before venturing outdoors.

pollens

In northern Europe, hay fever is seasonal, with the major triggers being grass pollens. The situation is more complex in America and Australia, where seasonal variations are less distinct and many pollens are airborne throughout the year.

There are certain plant species that seem particularly likely to trigger an allergic attack. These species include grasses, trees such as yew, oak, birch and willow, and flowers such as rose, wisteria, ragweed (a common trigger in North America), and ornamental lilies – especially the giant "star gazer" variety. Plants that appear to be unlikely to produce an allergic reaction include ivy, holly, foxgloves, hostas, hydrangeas and all herbs.

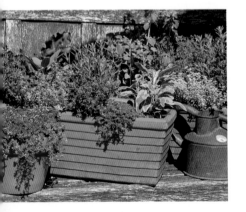

◀ *Herbs are attractive and useful plants and they are usually well tolerated by most hay fever sufferers.*

Take a walk over rolling hills, through woodland, along the beach, or in the mountains and breathe deeply. Feel your lungs fill up with fresh, clean air, and life-giving oxygen.

self-help

If you have a chronic breathing problem, an allergy or intolerance, or even just a temporary cold, there are many simple and practical measures you can take to look after yourself.

Our quality of life has a profound effect on the health of our lungs, and for better breathing, the best long-term strategy is a healthy lifestyle. This involves taking regular exercise, having enough sleep and eating a balanced diet. It is vital to strike a good balance between work and relaxation and to take care of our emotional needs. It is also important to maintain spiritual health, perhaps through meditation or prayer.

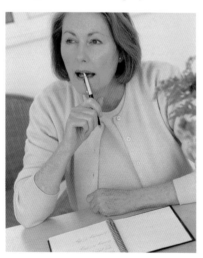

▲ *Keeping a diary can help pinpoint which substances may be triggering an allergy.*

the dangers of smoking

Tobacco smoke is responsible for 88 per cent of deaths from chronic lung disease, outweighing all other factors, including air pollution and occupational exposure to pollutants. It also weakens the immune system, and upsets the digestive system. Even if you don't smoke, "passive" or second-hand smoke is also a health hazard. So look after your lungs and stay away from smoky atmospheres; ask for a smoke-free zone in your local bar or restaurant, or choose places that already have one, and don't allow smoking in your home.

allergy awareness

For allergy-related breathing problems, always check labels for ingredients and additives. Keep a diary to pinpoint which substances may be causing an allergic reaction: perfumes, cosmetics, foods, pets, pollens and air pollution are all common triggers. Once you know what you are allergic to, you need to avoid it as far as possible, while also taking steps to build up your health and boost your immune system.

250 just relax

Many breathing problems have a psychological as well as a physical component. Anxiety, tension and worry are usually a contributory factor and so it is important to find ways to relax.

The profile of a typical asthmatic or allergy-sufferer is someone who is generally stressed, tense, hyperactive and hypersensitive. This creates constriction or tightness in the body's musculature and a feeling of being on "top note" all the time.

Finding time to unwind is important: when we are totally relaxed, our breathing slows and softens to an almost imperceptible whisper. We are also better able to cope when we are relaxed. There are many ways to relax, including taking exercise, meditating or soaking in a lavender-scented bath. Activities such as yoga and t'ai chi are also beneficial, as is spending "quality" time with friends and family.

DAILY TIPS FOR RELAXING
- take regular breaks when working
- enjoy walks in the fresh air
- don't skip meals
- don't "eat on the run"
- take a few deep breaths
- smile
- talk to a friend
- make time for yourself

lie down and relax
Find a few moments to lie down and relax by following these simple steps.

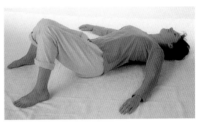

1 Roll up a towel and place it on the floor. Lie down with the towel along your spine with your knees bent and feet apart, allowing the head to drop back on to the floor or a thin pillow. The towel will help your chest to open.

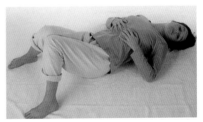

2 Place your fingers along the ribs, gently pressing into the muscle tissue as you breathe out. As the diaphragm relaxes, your breathing will start to deepen and relax.

index

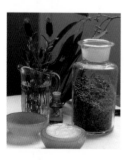

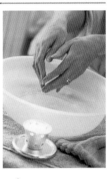

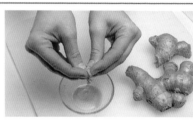

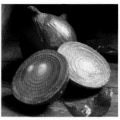